Praise

Our way of relating to food in contemporary culture has been twisted by fear, unmet needs for love, and the need to control. In this brilliant and groundbreaking book, you'll discover a powerful way to let go of "dieting" and awaken an intimate, intuitive connection with your body, mind, and spirit.

Tara Brach
Author of *Radical Acceptance* and *True Refuge*

With great insight and compassion, Heidi offers a way out of the common struggle with diet and weight. She supports her "10 steps" with a compelling blend of professional experience, personal experience, and scientific evidence that addresses not only our relationship with food but also our deep need for self-acceptance and a way of life that nurtures mind, body, and soul. Bravo!

Susan Kano
Author of *Making Peace with Food*

If you're looking for a book that will help you feel more sane and comfortable around food while learning to eat more nutritiously, Nourish *is an excellent choice. Heidi provides a blend of her personal recovery experience and professional and clinical wisdom that will guide you well on the road to recovery.*

Karen R. Koenig, MEd, LCSW
Author of seven books on improving eating and self-care

Heidi has met the challenge of putting her nutrition-counseling techniques into written form, allowing the ripples of her work to spread far beyond those lucky individuals who get to meet with her in person.

Jessica Setnick, MS, RD, CEDRD
Author of *The Eating Disorders Clinical Pocket Guide*
and Eating Disorders Boot Camp

I have read so many books on food, diet, and health, and I finally feel I can stop. Heidi's book reminds us that we are all unique and that, instead of looking for the "right" way to eat from the experts, all of the answers are actually inside ourselves. Our bodies know. This book is filled with great advice, real stories, and examples. Ultimately, Heidi is a reassuring guide, helping us find our way back to natural, healthy, intuitive eating.

Ingrid Kelada
Psychologist and author of *21 Days to Happiness*

Nourish *is full of tools to change one's relationship with food. But this book is about so much more. Heidi guides people to stop relentlessly trying again and again without experiencing change. She encourages people to step away from the roar of self-hatred and to step toward self-love. This book offers a motivating, realistic lens to change how you listen to your hunger (physically and emotionally) and to make choices that bring peace and nourishment. We can't live happily without our basic needs being met—being well fed and choosing healthy relationships, among other things.* Nourish *is like no other book I've read, and it is a gift to the health field and the world in general. Bravo.*

Hannah Saxe, LICSW
Therapist and Eating Disorder Specialist

Thank you, Heidi, for writing this important contribution to the field of nutrition therapy. This book provides a clear understanding of how our clients recover and, more importantly, offers the tools for anyone to begin their journey. This will be a nourishing staple for clinicians and clients alike. Bravo!

Lisa M. Pearl, MS, RDN, CEDRD-S
Certified Eating Disorders Specialist and Supervisor

This is a must-read for anyone working with people struggling with eating disorders or disordered eating. Heidi's own personal experience and honest examination of this topic are inspiring and very hopeful. So many of her statements about recovery will stick with me forever. Heidi walks people through the process of recovery in a non-critical manner and does this with ease. This book was a joy to read, and I will be recommending it to all of my clients.

Beth Mayer, LICSW
Executive Director of MEDA,
The Multi-Service Eating Disorders Association

Nourish speaks to the reader as Heidi speaks in person—with authenticity, playfulness, clarity, vulnerability, and, paramountly, with wisdom and respect. Heidi is a dancer and a storyteller at heart, as well as an artful nutrition therapist; her creative work with our shared clients has been a giant component in their stories of recovery. It is always a delight working alongside Heidi, and that sense of delight dances straight through the pages of Nourish. If you don't have the good fortune to work with Heidi live, then read her book because you get to not only drink in the bounty of her unique knowledge—you also get to take her home with you!

Lauren Manasse, LICSW, CEDS-S
Certified Eating Disorder Specialist and Supervisor

Nourish is the much-needed book that integrates the science of nutrition with holistic and attuned self-care. Heidi provides practical guidance on how to eat but within the context of intuitive self-knowledge. This is literally the only nutrition book I feel safe recommending to my clients. Thank you, Heidi!

Marci Evans, MS, CEDRD-S, LDN, cPT
Food and Body Image Healer™; Eating Disorders Expert

Nourish reaches out to hurting individuals on so many levels. It's not about eating disorders as much as it is about learning to unwind and reconnect with yourself so you can correctly interpret your own needs. It's about dismantling all of our preconceived ideas about what we should be like and learning to relax and become confident in who we are. This reaches beyond eating to so many other areas of life.

Nicole Spear, MS, CNS, CFMP
Certified Nutrition Specialist® Professional
Certified Functional Medicine Practitioner
Author of *Healthy Gut, Healthy Life*

This book is like a warm hug or a cool hand on your forehead when you're overheated with hating your tummy or your thighs, or thinking you're not good enough, for any reason. Heidi takes you by the hand and shows you how to eat for what your body really needs. As a nutrition therapist, and someone who suffered from the same issues she addresses, you can tell that Heidi knows what she's talking about and has helped many people in her practice. This awesome book is your opportunity to have Heidi help you. Buy a copy for every one of your friends who obsesses about her weight or body shape. She will thank you for it.

Lynda Goldman
Author of *Write to Heal*

nourish

how to heal your relationship with food, body, and self

HEIDI SCHAUSTER, MS, RDN, CEDRD-S

Nourish: How to Heal Your Relationship with Food, Body, and Self
Copyright © 2018 by Heidi Schauster
Hummingbird Press, Somerville, MA
Printed in the United States of America
Cover and Interior: 1106 Design

Publisher's Cataloging-In-Publication Data
(*Prepared by The Donohue Group, Inc.*)
Names: Schauster, Heidi.
Title: Nourish : how to heal your relationship with food,
body, and self / Heidi Schauster, MS, RDN, CEDRD-S.
Description: Somerville, MA : Hummingbird Press,
[2018] | Includes bibliographical references.
Identifiers: ISBN 9780999512005 (paperback) | ISBN 9780999512012 (ebook)
Subjects: LCSH: Food habits--Psychological aspects. | Compulsive eating--
Psychological aspects. | Self-esteem. | Mind and body. | Nutrition.
Classification: LCC TX357 .S38 2018 (print) | LCC TX357 (ebook) | DDC 613.2--dc23

Library of Congress Control Number: 2018934537

For information about this title or to order books in quantity, contact the author directly:
Heidi Schauster, MS, RDN, CEDRD-S
Nourishing Words Nutrition Therapy
617-877-2202
http://anourishingword.com
heidi@anourishingword.com

*Please do not substitute material in this book for actual consultation with a registered dietitian/
nutritionist, or mental-health clinician. The information presented in this book is not meant
as a specific treatment recommendation or personal communication with any individual,
nor should it replace any professional or medical advice. This publication is designed to
provide accurate and authoritative information regarding the subject matter covered to the
best of our knowledge. It is sold with the understanding that the publisher is not engaged in
rendering psychological, financial, legal, or other professional services. If medical care, expert
assistance, or counseling is needed, the services of a competent professional should be sought.
The author and publisher disclaim all liability in connection with the use of this book.*

Table of Contents

INTRODUCTION   Food Is Love (But Don't Eat Too Much)—Why This Mixed Message Hurts ix

STEP 1   Ditch Dieting for Good. 1

STEP 2   Body Acceptance, If Not Love 15

STEP 3   Awareness Before Action 35

STEP 4   Body Trust and Deep Listening. 55

STEP 5   Mindful Eating with Nutritional Common Sense 77

STEP 6   Conscious, Joyful Movement 105

STEP 7   Clarify Values to Live a Life You Love 121

STEP 8   Sustaining Self-Care Practices. 141

STEP 9   Developing a Self-Connected Eating Style . . . 159

STEP 10   Know the Company You Keep: Building a Support Tribe. 191

Introduction

Food Is Love (But Don't Eat Too Much)—Why This Mixed Message Hurts

W hen most of us were newborn infants, food was indeed love. We simply asked for what we needed. We cried. If our caregivers were tuned in, we got fed. You may have noticed that it's pretty hard to feed a baby—breast or bottle—without a comforting embrace. When the conditions are right, feeding and eating are truly one of the first times our needs are expressed and met as human beings. If you currently eat or withhold food to comfort yourself, you are not alone. You probably learned at a very young age that comfort and food are connected. In fact, food and love and caregiving are rather entwined. In its purest form, eating is a pleasure and feels good.

If you are reading this book, perhaps you feel that your relationship with food and your body is a bit out of whack.

When we stray with food, we often long to feel cared for but don't have the skills to ask for what we want. We want to be like that little baby, who simply cries when hungry and feeds at her mother's breast until she has had enough, drifting off to a sweet, satisfied sleep. As adults, we want and need to take breaks from our days to attend to our bodies, nourish them with food, and then return to our activities refreshed, fueled, and with new appreciation because we've paused to take the time to care for ourselves.

This kind of self-care is not an easy task when eating has become a mind-driven activity. And, yes, the very health and nutrition fields of which I am a part are at least partly to blame for us straying from that natural way of eating. We ask our minds instead of our bodies what they need. "What should I eat? What has the most nutrition? The least calories? The least carbs?" If you've ever stood agonizing over a menu, not knowing what the "right" choice is, you are not alone. Part of the problem is that we have so many food choices and so much health and nutrition information—often contradictory. We tend to use our minds to make food choices and leave our bodies out of the decision. Doing so takes us away from our innate capacity to feed ourselves well. We were born with that ability, but the diet and health industry—and all the other things in life pulling for our attention—steer us away from listening to that inner wisdom.

Before I struggled with my own eating, food was nourishing and tasty, and it felt good in my body. When I started to use food for other purposes as a teen—binge-eating to numb feelings or restrictive eating with the hope of changing my developing body—I lost the sweet, innocent, open relationship that I had with food in my childhood years. I was a perfectionist and a dancer who did not want to have a stomach full of dinner before my evening ballet classes. When I came home tired and hungry late at night, I was ravenous and overate. Then I felt terribly guilty and ashamed of my behavior. I eventually studied college nutrition and psychology and began to understand how my mind and body were out of balance. I began to see that not knowing how to fuel my young, active body had led me to food restriction, bulimia, and binge-eating.

I was very fortunate to stumble upon a lecture by Ellyn Satter at my university in 1992. I still have a signed copy of *Child of Mine: Feeding with Love and Good Sense*, her groundbreaking book on feeding children. In that lecture, I was blown away by her message: Listen to the body to decide what to eat. Having grown up in a Diet Pepsi culture, with almost daily ballet classes and the message that I needed to be careful not to eat too much or my stomach would not be so "dancer-ly," I was unused to making food decisions based on what I wanted to eat. My free and easy enjoyment of food as a child had turned into a head-based "should" kind of eating that was all about how to remain a svelte ballerina. And, of course, the more I dieted and tried to eat less, the more I slowed my metabolism and digestion, gained weight, encouraged binge-eating, and sapped my energy.

After hearing Ellyn Satter speak and meeting her in person, I was even more inspired to learn about the psychology of eating, not just about nutrition. It was a different track in nutrition school back in the early '90s. I knew I had found the path to finish healing my eating disorder, as well as a possible career in the area of eating-behavior change. I was lucky enough to continue to read books that were alternative at the time (*Intuitive Eating* by Evelyn Tribole and Elyse Resch, *Full Lives* by Lindsey Hall, *Making Peace with Food* by Susan Kano, and *When Women Stop Hating Their Bodies* by Jane Hirschmann and Carol Munter). These authors from the late '80s and '90s contradicted some of my other nutrition-science studies and suggested that dieting and trying to eat less, less, less might not be the way to health or well-being—never mind the "perfect" dancer's body. I learned more about the role that my struggle with food had in my life transition into adulthood. Over time, I developed a more accepting, loving relationship with my body and emerging self.

Over the last twenty-two years, I have worked with many clients who have also lost sight of the natural connection that food has to take care of body and self. Whether through over- or under-eating—or cycling between the two—so many of us lose the ability to trust our bodies to tell us what and how much to eat. Often a new acquaintance or client will ask, "Heidi, will you recommend a good basic book on nutrition for me to read?" I feel repeatedly stumped by that question. There are thousands of health and nutrition books out there. I often, in good faith, can't recommend them. Why? Because so many health and nutrition books are diet books in disguise—or they have messages that encourage dieting or controlling your food intake to achieve the desired outcome. There is no "basic" book that I can find that explains nutrition the way my colleagues and I do in practice—and does so in a way that I found so healing when I was recovering from disordered eating myself. I learned about nutrition and psychology not only as a way to obtain a college science degree, but also as a way to discover how to eat and fuel my body in a way that I'd never learned anywhere else.

How do we get back to this connected, embodied way of eating? My hope is that this book will assist you in re-learning to tune in—to your body, as well as your feelings, needs, and wants—so that you can make choices with food and other areas of self-care that are life-sustaining and supportive of your goals, dreams, and core values. Often, when our relationship to food and body feels out of alignment, other areas in our lives feel that way, too. This book has been born out of a deep desire in me to integrate work that I've done both personally and professionally. After witnessing so many people's journeys, I believe that healing our relationships with food and our bodies brings us to richer, fuller, and more meaningful lives. Care for yourself by consciously eating, mindfully moving your body, and building sustaining self-care practices and connections; it truly does set you free.

But it doesn't happen overnight, especially if you're out of practice or never actually learned to do this self-care in the first place. This book will give you a road map to finding that freedom. My hope is that *Nourish* reads like a conversation with someone you can trust to help you tune in to your own body's wisdom. As you can now well imagine, this is not going to be another diet book. If you want one of those, well, there's a whole section at your local bookstore. What I hope to offer you is an alternative that guides you through a journey of learning how to feed yourself well. There won't be any prescriptions here. There won't be lots of charts and lists of foods to eat or avoid. In fact, if you are tired of the diet roller coaster, on and off again with weight and food plans, this is the antidote for you. If you are recovering from an eating disorder, particularly in the later stages, when your behaviors around food are less dangerous but you still struggle with decisions about what to eat, then this is also written for you. If you are someone who feels like your relationship with food has gotten a little challenging over the years, then read on.

Eating, while something we often take for granted, is a learned behavior. And things can indeed go awry in the feeding or eating relationship. In 1996, I published an article based on some work that I did in graduate school with children who had multiple physical deformities and who had been fed through their stomachs by a gastric tube since birth.[1] These kids were typically born without use of their arms and legs. They struggled in their lives in so many ways. One of the areas was eating. These children had missed the natural windows in infancy and toddlerhood, when feeding cues happen and feeding progresses. They didn't need to learn how to eat because they had all of their nutritional needs met through the tube connected to their stomachs. As you can imagine, they didn't find food pleasurable at all, and many had aversions to having any food introduced into their mouths.

My colleagues and I worked with these children to investigate their fears around food and, for some, to eventually learn

---

[1] Schauster H. and Dwyer J. Transition from tube feedings to feedings by mouth in children: preventing eating dysfunction. *J Am Diet Assoc.* 1996;96(3):277-81.

to find pleasure in eating. We proposed a step-wise process to transition the children from tube-feeding to feeding by mouth. Some of the steps included establishing a positive relationship between feeder and child, oral stimulation and other work on the feeding environment, and eventually a progressive, behavioral feeding program. I still remember like it was yesterday the expressions on some of the kids' faces when they finally got past their fight-or-flight response to having food near their mouths. They started to enjoy the taste of something delicious for the first time.

I learned a lot from my time with these kids. They are, of course, an extreme example; but I do believe that all of our relationships with food develop out of our experiences and culture. When imbalanced, it takes intention, attention, and sometimes hard work to change our behaviors around food. The steps outlined in this book are quite different from the steps created in that child research long ago, but the result is the same: A healthier, more life-giving relationship with eating and its connection to the body and self.

What do you do if you've gotten so far away from a natural way of eating? What if you don't even know when you're hungry or full? Or what you want to eat? What if you only know how to choose the "safe" or lowest-calorie choice off of a menu, and it scares you to think of ordering what you *really* want? What if your relationship with food has been severely off-kilter, and you find yourself in a diet-binge cycle or feel terribly guilty after eating anything with sugar or carbohydrates? What if you want to have a more easeful, peaceful relationship with food, but it doesn't feel possible? After all, you grew up around dieters or were put on your first diet when you were ten. Or maybe you now read all the nutrition blogs and see the happy, healthy-looking, beautiful people who must know how to eat better than you do. Instead, I offer you a non-prescriptive, non-diet, body-accepting approach to healing your relationship with food.

The next ten chapters or Steps are not meant to be linear. I've put the Steps in a certain order because it's a progression that made sense to me and that seems to play out in my work with clients. They are meant to be fluid, liquid steps—not fixed or rigid. They were certainly cornerstones in my own journey and for many who consider themselves to have worked on and obtained a healthy relationship with food. It doesn't mean that we don't struggle with self-compassion or body acceptance anymore. It means that we have ways to deal with issues when they come up instead of restricting, dieting, or overeating. It also doesn't mean that we never under- or overeat. We sometimes eat mindlessly or in an un-attuned way. When we do, we get curious—not critical—about it. We notice it happening, check in, learn from the episode of funky eating, and ultimately let it go.

The first chapter or Step 1 involves ditching dieting: The important foundational step of intuitive eating. Step 2 is about body acceptance. We will delve into the research-supported world of Health-At-Every-Size® (HAES®) and bust up the weight-loss mindset that so often wrecks our eating and takes us away from caring for our bodies well. Step 3 is about developing awareness of our relationship with food, and its challenges, before trying to change anything. Step 4 is about body trust. I describe mindfulness and practices for tuning in to hunger and fullness, and I discuss the role meditation can play in this process. Step 5 is a "meaty" chapter about mindful eating choices and nutritional common sense. Step 6 invites you in to conscious, joyful movement of your body. Step 7 delves into the Acceptance and Commitment Therapy (ACT) principle of values clarification. We will look closely at universal human needs and how we nourish our souls. Step 8 encourages us to build sustainable self-care practices and deal with stress. Step 9 involves developing a self-connected eating style. In this chapter, I'll talk about questions that often come up in my practice around vegetarianism, gluten, other food sensitivities or allergies, food addiction, and "clean" eating. Lastly, Step 10 encourages you to know the company that you keep and build a tribe of support around you during the healing and growing process.

My wish is that these steps will help guide you on your journey to balance and wellness. It is my desire that all people learn to identify their deepest needs, wants, and hungers and to feed themselves in such a way that they feel nurtured, loved, freed up, and ready to take on the world. You don't have to spend so much time agonizing about what to eat or not eat. But you do need to devote some time and attention to feeding yourself well, on many levels.

Of course, this book is not a substitute for the incredible healing power of therapeutic relationships and professional help. When someone comes to see me for individual or group nutrition-therapy work, they often have other team members: Psychotherapists, primary care providers, psychiatrists, yoga/movement/art therapists, naturopaths, etc. I encourage you to share your reading here with trusted care providers and bring this work into any personal health and wellness work you are already doing. The stories of many different people are here in these pages. I changed the names of the clients who honored me with their stories to protect their privacy. I also use the pronoun "she" a fair amount and sprinkle in a "he" here and there, to mirror the demographics of my practice. I have learned that gender isn't binary, so my aim is not to exclude you if you do not use these pronouns to identify yourself. I use them for ease of reading and apologize in advance for any challenge that my wording brings up for you. Problems with eating, body, and self know no boundaries and affect all of us.

Lastly, please read this book with a grain of sea salt. As with any advice from a health professional or other, assorted wisdom-imparting human beings, I invite you to take the information, exercises, and anecdotes to heart that work for you and leave the rest. You are in charge of your journey. (If you don't feel like you are in charge with food, well, we'll get to that shortly. Step 1 may help immensely, though it can be one of the hardest steps.) No one knows more about what you need than you do. I hope this book helps you get in touch with what truly nourishes *you* on so many levels.

STEP 1

Ditch Dieting for Good

Dieting is one of those busy activities that we engage in when we don't want to face our fears and discontents. It gives us the illusion that we are in control of our lives—or at least our waistlines.

~ Tara Brach in *Radical Acceptance*

The biggest seller is cookbooks, and the second is diet books—how not to eat what you've just learned how to cook.

~ Andy Rooney

T he diet industry is a roughly $60 billion industry. It's a thriving industry based on the fact that, most of the time, the diet doesn't work. When a diet isn't sustainable (and most restrictive food plans are not), we then look for the next diet book or product or program. Often we circle back to ones that worked in the short term, hoping that, this time, the weight loss will stick. Research shows that most people who go on a diet will gain the weight back, often plus more. A UCLA study determined that one of the best predictors of weight gain is having been on a diet in the past year. Other research indicates that four out of five American women are dissatisfied with the way they look, with half of them on a diet. By age eighteen, 80 percent of girls report that they have dieted at some point in their life. Going on a diet is a predictor for having an increased body weight, particularly if you went on a diet during your child or teen years. I tell prospective nutrition-therapy clients that I don't do weight-loss counseling in my practice because I feel that it's unethical. I don't even have a scale in my office.

What I can help people with is improving their relationship with food. I don't have a crystal ball that tells me where my clients' bodies will land when they shift the way they operate with food and develop a more natural, mindful way of eating. Some of them who have put on excess weight because of binge-eating (or cycling between dieting and overeating) do eventually lose weight when they stop dieting and manipulating their food choices. Not all of them do. Some people gain weight, and some stay the same. There are so many factors that affect body size and weight. Sometimes clients are on medications that affect their metabolism and weight, or they have thyroid conditions to address. Sometimes they are meant to be in a larger body size than they want to be and have to work on accepting their beautiful, large bodies in order to learn to feed them well. (More on this hard step in the next chapter.)

Step 1

Yes, I will assert that some people have to gain weight to find peace with food. In a culture that values thinness above all other body types right now, that can be challenging. But I promise you that letting go of weight loss as the outcome will bring you so much more freedom and vitality. Instead, focus on food, exercise, and self-care choices that feel health-enhancing. Weight loss (or gain, if one's tendency is to be underweight when unbalanced) is sometimes a side effect of the work, but it has to be a "back burner" goal. If you focus on eating in a balanced, healthful, life- and energy-sustaining way, I believe that your health and well-being will improve. My colleagues and I have worked with many clients in this non-weight-focused way with much success.

There is no denying that the desire to lose weight and be thinner often drives problematic eating behaviors. Eating disorders like anorexia nervosa (restrictive eating) and bulimia nervosa (binge/purge cycling) are prevalent and destructive. Eating disorders lead to more deaths than any other psychiatric disorder, so they are serious concerns that require treatment, ideally early on. I talked about my journey with an eating disorder in the Introduction of this book. Despite the emphasis on restrictive dieting in our culture, the most common eating disorder is Binge Eating Disorder (binge-eating without purging). A vast majority of these eating disorders are fueled—at least initially—by the desire to lose weight and feel in control. Eating disorders are more prevalent in developed countries where food is plentiful and the aesthetic ideal is thin.

Eating disorders are complex emotional disorders which are not just about diet and weight. Individuals with eating disorders are in a great deal of pain, and they are using food and their body to communicate that. The obsession with food and weight and the cycle of over- and under-eating can take on a life of its own. Even if you don't have a diagnosed eating disorder, you can have a complicated relationship with food. Perhaps that's why you are reading this book. Maybe you or a loved one is struggling with balance around food. There may be significant, underlying emotional struggles, but the diet-oriented and thin-obsessed culture that we live in fuels the fight.

If you fear and detest weight gain, you may not feed yourself well all day, only to find yourself binge-eating at night. If you wish to be thinner, you may make food choices that are about calories and not about your own body's wisdom about what it wants at that moment. Then you feel unsatisfied and find yourself looking for the cookies later. By focusing on weight loss—instead of balance, health, and nourishment—you may promote the very weight gain that you want to abolish. Ironically, trying to lose weight can keep you stuck in a struggle with food and your body.

There are many ways in which body weight is not determined by how much food we eat. Some of the ways are metabolism differences, heredity, hormones, and even something that I have learned about more recently, called "epigenetics." The short story on epigenetics around weight is this: The way your parents and grandparents ate during your and your mother's conception may affect your body weight and your tendency to be a particular body shape and size. No kidding. Most interestingly, a study of Dutch famine victims showed that parents who conceived children during this time of starvation went on to have children who were significantly higher weight than their siblings. It's as if these kids, whose pregnant mothers didn't have enough to eat, entered the world as caloric-energy conservers, ready for famine. Unfortunately, they then grew up in a world where food was abundantly available, and their genes couldn't adjust. I sometimes wonder if this isn't one of those less-discussed factors when we hear about the increased weight of each generation, the so-called "obesity epidemic." Could it be that dieting mothers and grandmothers (instructed to do so for health reasons, so they don't gain too much weight in pregnancy) are inadvertently putting their children at risk for the very "obesity" that they are trying to avoid? Fascinating—and yet another reason not to restrict calories during pregnancy!

So, maybe you are already working on trying not to diet or restrict your eating. If so, congratulations! It's a super-hard part of the process for some. Even if you feel you are there, the culture of dieting may try to suck you back in. The latest diet disguised as "clean" eating may fool you. Your Aunt Margaret and her new way of eating that gives her so much more energy may fool you. Remember that the wealthy diet industry is well marketed and based on the fact that people will come back to it when it doesn't work. The diet industry tells you that, left to your own devices, you'd be out of control. I don't believe this for a second. Learning to trust your body and its wisdom is part of the process of learning to feed yourself well. (We'll get there in more depth in Step 4.) Don't let another diet or health guru tell you that you can't be trusted!

When I work with someone who has had decades of struggles around food and weight, we often trace it back to that first time she got put on a diet—either by herself, a family member, or even by a well-meaning doctor. Often, my clients look back sadly and say, "I wasn't even really heavy back then. I would love to get back to that weight! Why did I think I was too fat then?" Unfortunately, yo-yo dieting wreaks havoc on metabolism, not to mention on self-esteem. When you consciously try to eat less, especially when you restrict your food considerably, you lower your metabolism. The body needs those calories (our fuel, our gasoline) to run efficiently.

If we don't get enough calories to meet our needs, we don't just drop dead (at least not right away); the body just does what it does slower. That's why many chronic restrictive dieters have irritable bowel and constipation on their problem list—slow-digestion problems. Those with severe anorexia nervosa have dangerously slow heart rates. Restrictive dieters' hair might get thinner, and their menstrual periods might stop. When we're not eating enough, our hearts keep beating, and our brains keep functioning. The calories go to the vital body functions, but they don't go to the not-so-vital ones, like hair or fertility or keeping us warm.

Dieters often feel colder than everyone around them, or foggy in the head, or exhausted and fatigued all of the time. The diet industry wants you to believe that's all about sugar or gluten or something else that you should eliminate. Food sensitivities (which we'll visit in Step 9) are real for some people, but I can't tell you how many times symptoms of sluggishness, fatigue, lack of focus, and slow digestion go away when clients simply start eating more food—*any* food, and *especially* carbohydrates, which diet culture vilifies. (More on carbs in Step 5.)

I love Rebecca Scritchfield's podcast, of the same name as her book, *Body Kindness*. Rebecca is a registered dietitian nutritionist with a Health-At-Every-Size approach to her work. She interviews guests on topics that help listeners create better well-being and heal their relationships with their bodies. The podcast includes regular chats with her friend, Bernie Salazar. He is a former contenstant from the popular reality TV show *The Biggest Loser*, which was canceled in February 2016. Bernie was the at-home "winner" of season 5, and he received the runner-up prize money. Like other contestants, he dieted and exercised excessively to lose weight. Like most other former contestants, Bernie gained the weight back. (Notice that the show didn't follow the dieters over the long-term.)

Bernie is now approaching his relationship to health differently, with balance and respect for his body for the rest of his life. Bernie can't work out umpteen hours per day, like he had to do on the show, and still live the life that he wants to lead—but he can eat well and exercise regularly. He is finding the balance that works for him physically, mentally, and emotionally. It's an inspiring podcast, and I recommend that you check it out if you are struggling to let go of dieting yourself. Rebecca and Bernie are using an intuitive-eating and mindful-movement perspective that you will read my version of here in Steps 5 and 6.

We just looked at the ways dieting affects the body; now let's explore the way dieting affects the mind. I recently reviewed a study with colleagues that looked at whether people associated the word "celebration" or "guilt" with chocolate cake. It's probably no surprise that the people who picked "guilt" had more problematic behaviors around food. Those who chose "celebration" when they thought of chocolate cake had a more easeful relationship with food. The interesting finding is that those who picked "guilt" also seemed to struggle more with losing weight (when they wanted to) versus those who chose "celebration." The authors of the study were trying to demonstrate what so much other research—and my personal and work experience—has shown: "Diet thinking" doesn't work and can actually promote weight gain over time.

When I speak to parent groups, I often tell them that I can turn any of their children into a binge-eater. Parents are then all ears because they do not want a child who binges and reaches a higher body weight any more than they themselves want to be stigmatized by our culture for their own habits and body. I tell them that the single-most surefire way to make their child a binge-eater is to take away all their favorite foods. For when those foods become forbidden, they become more attractive, more charged. A cookie is just a cookie if you can have it anytime you want one. And, yes, kids are able to eat cookies moderately. But if you paint a picture of scarcity and say that cookies are forbidden or restrict them to only particular times, they then become more charged. They become cookies with a capital "C."

Yes, this works with grown-ups and food, too. When we're on a diet, there is often a very young part of us that is itching to rebel against the restriction. **Internal Family Systems (IFS) is** a branch of psychotherapy that investigates the different parts of us that may be in operation at any given time. This rebellious young part in many of us does not like to be deprived and wants the cookies even more now that they are forbidden. It's human nature to want what we can't have.

It's also human nature to want to control things when our lives feel a little chaotic—or a lot chaotic. But trying to control food is a recipe for chaos. The mind wants what it can't have even more. And when the body is starving, the drive to eat and think about food all the time increases. Also, the digestive hormone ghrelin gets secreted when we are emptier than our bodies would like us to be. Ghrelin makes us feel even more hungry. It's the body's natural weight regulator and tells us it's time to eat. So, when dieting, we have all of these forces working against the diet. No wonder it's so hard to eat less food sustainably! In Step 5, we'll look at why focusing on self-care when making food choices—instead of self-control—is the answer to eating in a way that supports a healthy relationship with our bodies.

Let's summarize the physical and psychological risks of dieting, beyond the tendency to regain the weight and develop a challenging relationship with food:

Physical risks of repeated dieting include:

- Poor nutrition and nutrient deficiencies

- Slow metabolism and digestion

- Fatigue

- Weakness

- Hypertension

- Increased risk of cardiac and cardiovascular problems

- Premature aging with weight cycling and poor nutrition
- Gallstones

Psychological risks of repeated dieting include:

- Obsession with weight
- Heightened responsiveness to external food cues
- Decreased enjoyment of food
- Disordered eating patterns
- Disordered lifestyle (excessive or inadequate exercise, social life affected by avoiding certain eating occasions, etc.)
- Increased incidence of eating disorders
- Increased pressure to conform to society's standards of beauty
- Increased sense of failure
- Decreased self-esteem
- Financial burden

So, if dieting doesn't work (the roughly 95 percent chance you'll gain the weight back is just not good odds), then what is the alternative if you want to feel good in your body at the beach this summer? Well, first and foremost, remember to view yourself as a whole person (body, mind, and spirit—not just body), and take care of *all* of you. We'll talk about accepting—and maybe even loving—our amazing, miraculous bodies in the next chapter, Step 2. If you have a troubled relationship with your body and with food, finding a way to nourish your body with balance and care can be a struggle.

What is a non-diet way of maintaining your own healthy body weight, no matter what body type you were born with?

Non-diet eating involves:

- Listening to what the body needs

- Responding to internal cues of hunger instead of external cues (sight, smell, the power of suggestion) most of the time

- Not turning to food to deal with stress

- Being personally in charge of food choices instead of being controlled by a diet prescription

- Realizing that feeling healthy and taking good care of your body will make you more attractive than a diet will

- Abandoning short-term weight loss for long-term and lasting self-confidence, health, and wellness

- Having space for more nourishing pursuits and for what matters in life

You choose your path, but I hope I've given you enough reasons to ditch demoralizing dieting for good. **Remember that it's not that you don't have willpower. Don't let the wealthy diet industry convince you of that. You have the**

power and control and choice to take the best care of your body that you can. Dieting might be making you feel like a failure. Restrictive eating is not sustainable. Our bodies and minds protect us against it by making us want and need to eat. And eat more.

Do your body and spirit a favor, and throw out the diet (and maybe even the string bikini that you wore when you were eighteen and you swear that you will get into again some day). Respect your body where it's at, and help it ease into the healthiest shape that it can be by vowing never to diet again. And if you need help with a troubled relationship with food, my colleagues and I who do this non-diet kind of nutrition therapy would be happy to help you practice tuning in, listening, and respecting that inner wisdom that we all have within us. Most of us used to eat intuitively and according to our bodies' needs when we were young—until the diet industry and other well-meaning persons told us that they know better. Learn to trust your own inner wisdom again instead. And until you can, I encourage you to find professionals to work with who believe in your body's wisdom.

The rest of the steps that follow in this book are designed to help you on the journey. As I mentioned before, they aren't meant to be linear. You will probably have to revisit Step 1 many times, as you catch yourself making food choices for diet-y reasons. The next step, Body Acceptance, is also not an easy one, but it's a vital step in the process toward a healthy, loving relationship with food and your whole self.

Step 1: References and Resources

Painter, R.C., Roseboom, T.J., Bleker, O.P. "Prenatal exposure to the Dutch famine and disease in later life: An overview." *Reproductive Toxicology.* 2005; 20: 345-352.

Kuijer, R.G. and Boyce, J.A. "Chocolate cake: Guilt or celebration? Associations with healthy eating attitudes, perceived behavioural control, intentions and weight-loss." *Appetite* 2014; 74: 48-54.

Bacon, L. and Aphramor, L. *Body Respect: What Conventional Health Books Get Wrong, Leave Out, and Just Plain Fail to Understand about Weight.* Dallas, TX: BenBella Books, Inc., 2014.

Scritchfield, R. *Body Kindness.* New York, NY: Workman Publishing Co., Inc., 2016.

Satter, E. *Secrets of Feeding a Healthy Family: How to Eat, Raise Good Eaters, How to Cook.* Madison, WI: Kelcy Press, 2008.

Schwartz, R.C. *Introduction to the Internal Family Systems Model.* Oak Park, IL: Trailheads Publications, 2001.

Sweezy, M. and Ziskind, E. *Innovations and Elaborations in IFS Therapy.* New York, NY: Routledge, 2017.

STEP 2

Body Acceptance, If Not Love

Perfectionism is defined as the compulsive need to achieve and accomplish one's goals, with no allowance for falling short of one's ideals. Perfectionists experience enormous stress and anxiety about getting things exactly right and then feel devastated when they don't. The unrealistically high expectations of perfectionists mean that they will inevitably be disappointed. By seeing things in black-and-white terms—either I'm perfect or I'm worthless—perfectionists are continually dissatisfied with themselves.

~ Kristin Neff, PhD, in *Self-Compassion*

In Step 1, I mentioned that the United States alone has a $60 billion diet industry. It also has approximately 6 to 11 million people with eating disorders. I think our Western culture has a bit of a perfectionism problem, particularly as it relates to thinness. As a recovering perfectionist myself, I can relate. The black-and-white thinking that Kristin Neff describes in the quote above drives us to work harder than our bodies and minds can take. It motivates us to live the perfect life, strive for the perfect body, eat the perfect food, and do the perfect exercises to get there. But what if our health and well-being were not so black-and-white?

Surprise! They aren't. Do you know someone who has lived a long life with a seemingly healthy body and not done tons of vigorous exercise or health-conscious eating? I do. My grandfather always kept moving. He was an engineer, carpenter, and golfer. He didn't sit around when one of his grandkids had a science-fair project to work on, but he never went to the gym. He was also Italian and grew up knowing and loving good food. He ate well but moderately: Meat, potatoes or pasta, vegetables, desserts some of the time. He liked food but never agonized about it. When his health failed in his later years, it tended to be during times when eating enough was a struggle. Oh, and he had a martini many evenings. Again, moderation. I never once saw him drunk as a skunk, but he liked to have his one drink. He lived to a ripe old age of ninety-seven. And while all the young guys were using golf carts, he would still walk the golf course into his early nineties. His wife, now ninety-four and living independently in the same house with regular visits from family, still says, "If you don't move it, you'll lose it."

I use the example of Grampy because he lived a long, healthy, active life without stressing so much about his health, body, or diet. In fact, there's some evidence that stress can have a bigger impact on health and weight gain than grandma's cheesecake—or, in the case of our family, Nana's mud pie. In Step 8, we will visit the topic of stress in much more depth.

One of the best ways to accept our bodies is to understand that there are so many forces at work that affect our body size, shape, and health. I mentioned in the last chapter (Step 1) that there are lots of reasons that we have the body shape and size that we do—reasons that have nothing to do with how we eat. Heredity, hormones, and lifelong physical-activity patterns (including how naturally mobile and fidgety or grounded and still you are) have a profound effect on your body size and shape. In the last chapter, I also mentioned epigenetics and the research that points to your mother's or grandmother's eating habits while pregnant as affecting your body weight.

Let's consider letting go of the myth that we need to live up to the body shape that is the cultural favorite of the day. I'm going to specifically talk here about women, though I am aware that our cultural biases towards thinness and perfection do, indeed, affect persons of all genders. From here on in, for ease of writing, I will use a binary distinction, "woman," knowing well that gender is not a binary construct for many people.

Many non-Western cultures today view female fatness as a sign of health, wealth, and vitality. Before the 1800s, so did Americans. In colonial days in the U.S., the voluptuous figure was generally seen as more desirable. Signs advertising weight-gain tonics were on display. In the 1900s (some say the 1920s flappers started it; some say Twiggy in the 1960s), we significantly shifted our aesthetic appreciation of women's bodies, and the media began to show thinner, lithe figures as the ideal. At the same time, the growing diet industry sold us the belief that we could do something to our bodies to live up to that thinner ideal. Feminist scholars highlight the rise of thinness and diet culture alongside the rise of women's liberation. Many believed it to be a backlash and response to the emerging power and equality of women, feared by the patriarchal structure of society. If this topic interests you, Naomi Wolf wrote about it at length in her popular book *The Beauty Myth*.

As food became more plentiful and mass produced, and as dieting for health and weight loss gained popularity, we started to recognize eating disorders as different and distinct physical- and mental-health issues. As I mentioned earlier, eating disorders occur in 6 to 11 million people in the United States alone—and that reflects only the statistics for those who actually report the disordered eating. If someone feels bad about her body and feels that she must be smaller than who she is in the present, then she is more likely to go on a diet. She is also liable to make food choices that reflect restriction rather than pleasure, exercise to exhaustion and not for enjoyment, and walk around with a general sense of being defective and too much.

Sometimes negative body feelings are beyond cultural comparisons and may stem from violation of the body by sexual or physical abuse or by a history of neglect of one's bodily or emotional needs. Sometimes there are issues around diverse sexual identity or gender (LGBTQ). What one cannot yet express may get displaced in body or eating issues. When any negative body thoughts—and the behaviors that stem from them—become constant, obsessive, and distracting from the rest of life, then an eating disorder may develop. Examples of this are Anorexia Nervosa, Bulimia Nervosa, Binge-Eating

Disorder (BED), or what we call Other Specified Feeding and Eating Disorder (OSFED). I find that most of the people I work with fit into the latter category.

Eating disorders are the number-one killer of all of the psychiatric illnesses. It is seriously dangerous for children, adolescents, and adults to go down this path. Despite this reality, bad body talk is somehow acceptable in our society. How many times have you overheard a bunch of women criticize their bodies as if this were a way to bond? Yuck. I don't believe it's an accident that eating disorders mainly occur in developed countries. In places where food is not plentiful and survival beats out body-sculpting for the typical pastime, obsession over food and body just doesn't exist. Eating disorders are complex problems that are about so much more than food and chasing body perfection, but we can't ignore the cultural context in which they flower. In this culture, we use our bodies and food as a way to express pain, neglect, sadness, anger, trauma, and a sincere desire (in all of us) to be loved and accepted.

I am often saddened and struck by the crippling negative body talk of my clients. In fact, if we look around, we hear it all over. It's as if it is entirely reasonable to bash our bodies at every turn.

"This makes me look fat."
"Oh, she's really let herself go ..."
"I probably shouldn't eat this. I'm too fat already."

And, the seemingly complimentary, but just as vicious ...

"Oh, you look so good! Did you lose weight?"

Somehow, our moral fabric gets attached to our body shape and size. These comments, while innocent at first glance, can be demoralizing. In fact, some of my clients have comments like these going on in their heads so much all day that it's hard for them to focus on much else. Others may be able to challenge those thoughts and function well in their lives but still feel a debilitating sense of shame and disgust around their bodies that percolates in the background.

Why do we pick on ourselves so much? Why do we narrowly see one body type as ideal and strive to fit into that mold? Why is "fat-ism" so prevalent? I'm not going to answer these questions adequately, because they aren't easy to answer in full. Yes, Marilyn Monroe's 1950s size 12 would be unacceptable in a decade where there is now a size 00. (Don't even get me started on that one!) Yes, the beauty industry insists on making us feel bad about our appearance by airbrushing pores, photo-shopping thighs, and giving us a picture of human beings that is downright fake. After all, if we felt excellent about ourselves, then we probably wouldn't buy that face cream or lipstick or diet product.

Subtle comments about weight to a "chubby" child go destructively deep and erode self-esteem. I hear about this childhood shame in the stories of so many of my clients who struggle with a challenging relationship with food for decades. Negative body thoughts (who doesn't have them sometimes?) can go awry and become the foundation on which develops a terrible relationship with eating and fitness. For some, this may ultimately lead to an eating disorder. Perhaps you are reading this book because you've struggled with disordered eating or because you just want to have a more peaceful relationship with

food and body. **I invite you to reframe how you talk to your-self (and those around you) about body weight and shape.**
I work with beautiful—truly beautiful, inside and out—people of all genders who do not like their bodies and themselves. These are successful, smart, funny, articulate, creative, and uniquely gifted individuals—but they cannot see it because all they see is how fat they are. It doesn't matter how much they weigh, either. They can be "underweight" or "overweight" according to the medical charts; what matters most is that they feel less than their full selves because of the way their bodies look. Does this sound like you?

What happens when negative body thoughts (again, who doesn't have them at least once in a while?) go all wrong? How does this thinking get out of control and develop into eating disorders for some and not others? There are so many factors—genetic, temperamental, and environmental among them—that predispose some people to eating disorders. What I've noticed frequently is that problematic eating and bad body thoughts become a way to take feelings that something is just not right and make them concrete. "I don't like myself" becomes easier to articulate if she says, "I don't like my body." "Something is not right in my life," becomes "Something is not right with my body."

If we don't like our bodies, the internet says that we can do all kinds of things to change them. It's an area of our lives that we can really have control over. But all the green smoothies and CrossFit in the world won't make us like ourselves any more, or compensate for painful feelings that we need to express, or make what feels wrong about our lives go away. The diet industry likes to feed us the image that if we just change our bodies, we can feel good and change our lives, but it's really not that simple.

Some of my clients "lose the weight" and realize that they don't feel much better about themselves. How devastating to find out that losing weight is never the answer to lifelong happiness! If it is, well, they often realize that it's a pretty shallow life that their deeper, truer selves aren't so interested in living. Now, mind you, I'm not bashing real self- and body-care. I'm a nutritionist, after all, and a dancer. I believe in taking good care of our amazing, capable vessels that bless us in our lifetimes. I believe in the body as one of our modes of self-expression. I work on helping my clients come to an appreciation of the beautiful part of us that the body is. However, our bodies are just *one part* of who we are. I might make a body connection when I dance with a partner—and that's lovely—but it's the people I make heart-and-soul connections with who nourish me on a deep level and keep me dancing with others.

Loving our bodies starts, in my opinion, and in my practice, with loving ourselves and with seeing our bodies as an extension of that self-love. I want to challenge you— whether you struggle with disordered eating or not—to ask yourself the following questions when you say something negative (out loud or in your mind) about your body. Ask yourself, "How am I feeling?" and "What's really not feeling good right now?"

Try it. Are those bad body thoughts coming up because you feel inadequate after talking to someone you admire? Are they coming up because you are feeling judged by a family member? Are you "feeling fat" because your dieting friend is ordering the burger without a bun, and you wonder if you should, too? Or are you "feeling fat" because you just ran up the stairs and feel more breathless than you did last week? "Fat" is, of course, actually not a "feeling." It's tougher to get in touch with other, deeper feelings of shame, inadequacy, fear, loneliness, exhaustion, and grief that might be under those negative body thoughts. The body is a great container for our negative energy.

When you feel bad about your body and ask yourself the question, "What's really going on right now?" you may get to what you are feeling in the present moment. When you do so, you may be less likely to use food (over- or under-indulgence) or exercise in a way that is self-destructive. You may, with practice over time, be able to substitute the destructive eating behavior (binge-eating or consciously going hungry, for example) with something that more adequately addresses the feelings underneath. Some of my clients have noticed, after careful reflection, that they use food restriction, binge-eating, purging, or hyper-exercise as a self-punishment. They really do feel terrible about themselves, and these behaviors make their internal struggle concrete and real—in real time. They **embody** their pain.

Once you notice what might be behind your negative body thoughts and eating behaviors, examine what doesn't feel right—either on your own or with a trusted friend or therapist. Don't succumb to body bashing just because it's socially accept-able. **We can't even begin to take good care of the bodies that we have if we hate them or if we loathe the person within.** I don't find that clients can make a lot of headway in their nutrition therapy or build and sustain self-care practices if they are also not doing the work of understanding and caring for their deeper, unique selves.

Please don't allow negative body thoughts to swim about in your head. Don't stay on the surface and say that you'd be happy "if only …" (insert transformative body change here). Question those negative thoughts! I invite you to be curious about them. Listen to what they tell you is wrong in your life. Don't be afraid to squirm when you discover the answers. And don't be afraid to ask for help. It's worth examining some painful truths to eventually come to a place of body acceptance and self-love.

Body acceptance takes time, especially if you've hated your body for decades. I promise you, though, that if you eat from a place of self-love and not self-control, you will indeed eat in a way that nourishes your body and nurtures your whole self. So, how to begin?

First, I recommend that you drop the scale (perhaps down a few flights of stairs) and focus on Health-At-Every-Size. HAES is a movement. (Really. Google it.) It's time for all of us to stop hating our bodies and accept the research. Health is not determined by weight but by habits, genes, and environment. I highly recommend Linda Bacon and Lucy Aphramor's book *Body Respect* if you need more help with this. They repeatedly cite research showing that weight and health are not as connected as our mainstream media would make us believe. Back in 2002, I heard Glenn Gaesser, PhD, speak about his book *Big Fat Lies: The Truth About Your Weight and Your Health.* It rocked my world as a registered dietitian/nutritionist, and I vowed never to do weight-loss counseling again. Dr. Gaesser went step by step through the "obesity research" studies and showed that, when controlling for the health effects of physical activity, the effect that weight has on health actually goes away.

Weight's role in health is exaggerated. Really. The reason that research studies (and reporters in the mainstream media) so often connect the two is that the *habits* often associated with those who happen to be in the highest weight categories (eating beyond fullness, eating outside of hunger, sedentary lifestyle, etc.) do, indeed, affect health. It's the *habits and not the weight* that are the problem. There are statistical ways to control different factors in research. Again, when most studies control for physical activity, the effect that weight has on health goes away. So, yes, you can be fat and fit and have a longer, healthier, more vibrant life than a skinny couch potato. Despite all the news coverage of the "war on obesity," the Centers for Disease Control in 2005 determined that only when the Body Mass Index (BMI) reaches 35+ is there a meaningful increase in mortality. People in the "overweight" (BMI 25–30) category actually have the longest lifespan. Why are we calling these people "overweight" anyway?

Don't believe the hype. Thin is not buying you any more disease-free years, particularly if your body is not naturally conditioned to be thin. What it does get you is a lifetime of obsessing that limits your ability to be really present in your relationships and life. No one said it better than Rachel Zimmerman, staff writer for WBUR, Boston's National Public Radio news station. Her article appeared first on WBUR's CommonHealth blog, and I reposted it on my own blog in December 2014. The article is entitled, "I'm Finally Thin—But Is Living in a Crazymaking Food Prison Really Worth It?"

"Thin privilege" is real in this culture. I know I have it. I occasionally have a brave client who says, "How can you know what it feels like to be very large and oppressed in this culture?" She's right; I don't. No amount of reading about size discrimination allows me to wear the shoes of someone who is living it. Once I recovered from my eating disorder in my twenties and settled into a more intuitive, mindful way of eating and physical activity, my body dropped the weight that came on through binge-eating and purging (myth-buster: purging does not keep your weight low). My body settled into the shape that I had before my eating disorder. Every year, I go to the doctor and get weighed for my physical (that's the only time I step on a scale), and my weight is always unremarkably the same and has been for about two decades. That is, except for the time when I was carrying and nursing twin daughters and gained nearly half my body weight. (I got to try on the voluptuous look for a bit and loved it.) If you don't fight with your body by dieting, your body will decide the healthiest weight for it. If you jump into dieting to "lose the baby weight," you begin the struggle and make it more likely that your body will want to hold on to that weight to protect you from the self-induced famine.

I have countless clients who, once embracing a more natural, intuitive way of eating, find they settle into a place where their bodies comfortably want to be—and they just stay there year after year. Some of them end up with lower weights than they initially were trying to maintain with their diet regimes; some of them end up with higher weights. Some have no change in their body weight at all but feel more vitality, energy, and acceptance. Grace is a client who has been making progress recovering from a pattern of restrictive eating alternating with binge-eating. She's been eating more intuitively and feeling good about herself, focusing more on her relationship with food instead of her weight. Then she goes in for a doctor's appointment and has to step on the scale. *Bam!* Her body and weight concerns quadruple, and she starts to doubt all the real progress she has been making. Then, perhaps not coincidentally, she finds a pair of jeans in her closet that don't fit anymore and tries to pour herself into them. The bad body thoughts skyrocket.

Now, why would she do that to herself? Why sink back into a place of body loathing when she has been working so hard on body acceptance? I wondered along with her, out loud, if being confident, self-assured, and asking for what she needs (from food, from anybody) is just less familiar than feeling bad. She knows she doesn't enjoy focusing on what she doesn't like about her body, but there is some sick kind of comfort in it. So many clients make progress and start to feel great about themselves; then they pull out those skinny jeans that no longer fit. Just this act puts them right back in a place of self-loathing, judgment, and feeling "less than."

When I talked to Grace about her resistance to telling the doctor not to weigh her (when the particular appointment had nothing to do with her weight) or donating the ill-fitting jeans, she admitted that she is afraid that she needs the scale and the jeans to "keep herself in check." If she doesn't have the jeans in her closet, she might "let herself go." Exploring further, she admits to worrying that, if she asks for what she needs, she will be "too much" and her needs will be too great. In her inner world, it's better to be small, not needy, more in control.

How many women worry about taking up too much space, needing too much, being too demanding or too "big"? Well, a lot of us do—and it's not just women. Grace was willing to let the jeans decide if she was good enough, despite all the work that she had been doing on her personal growth. It was another turning point in Grace's recovery when she finally gave me the skinny jeans that she had been trying on daily as a gauge of how she was doing. If she fit into them, it was a "good day," and she could eat in a more relaxed way; if she didn't, it was a "bad day," and she needed to restrict her food more. This created a roller coaster of under- and overeating and kept her obsessed with food. It also meant that those jeans were determining many of her daily actions and feelings. She was no longer wearing the pants in her life; the pants were wearing her (and wearing her out).

On a hot summer day, another client, Jennifer, said that she'd rather sweat in pants than show her legs in shorts. Where is the self inside that body? Could she come out and be heard? (She's hot in there, and she wants you to take care of her!) Do you measure your self-worth with a scale or a pair of skinny jeans or some other item of clothing? Or are you trying to "stay small" in your life by not needing much? Might you be battling with your natural body weight—or not even sure what your natural body weight is because you've fluctuated up and down so much?

Wouldn't it be fantastic if all of us put on that bathing suit and said, "Oh, look. I put on a little winter weight this year. Well, by the time I need to wear this, it'll fit. If not, I'll find a new one" and then just let nature take its course? I live in New England, where there are defined seasons. I naturally gravitate toward heavier foods in winter and lighter foods in summer. I also move less in the winter and get outside more in the warmer months. Many people freak out about this natural change in body with the seasons and diet like crazy in April and May. They often end up experiencing unhealthy weight-cycling. Many of my clients struggle each year with food in the spring, instead of just noticing the ebbs and flows of weight that just happen. Some women feel stress every month when their weight goes up predictably before their period, due to premenstrual bloating. I wish for them—and you—to know the truth: Deep down you are the same beautiful person, despite weight fluctuations.

We all want to feel good in our bodies. We all want to have vitality and strength and lightness of being. Putting too much emphasis on whether or not we can fit into a pair of jeans or a summer dress is a recipe for low self-esteem and a troubled relationship with food and exercise. I will challenge you the way I challenge many of my clients and blog readers every spring: Take everything in your closet that doesn't fit you, and donate it, consign it, or give it to a friend who will wear it. Why do we hold on to these things (anything, actually) that make us feel less than the stellar beings that we are? Wear things that make you feel good, express something about you, and always remember that you are so much more than the size of your clothes. We all know that a pretty house is delightful, but that alone doesn't make a happy home.

The bottom line: We will settle in at a weight that is right for our unique body and lifestyle when we stop bullying ourselves with restrictive eating, dieting, overeating, and compulsive exercising. **The only way to let go of the dieting mentality and the idea that our bodies need to change is by accepting that there is nothing wrong with them in the first place.** There may be some habits around food and movement that could be tweaked to become more self-loving. There may be some ways that we can manage stress more effectively to support our health and well-being. But, first, we must accept our bodies as they are. Right now. In this moment. We need to stop saying, "I'll start living when I lose x pounds." We need to start living *now*. It's a leap of faith to say, 1) "I'm not going to diet anymore," and 2) "I'm not going to look hatefully upon my body anymore." That's why I am putting these two Steps up front, even though I know you will revisit them over and over on the journey toward peace with food.

I honestly believe—and I've seen this over and over again in practice—that we can't change our habits in a long-lasting way if we are beating ourselves up in the process. We'll talk more about that in the next chapter, Step 3. Letting go of dieting and restricting and coming into harmony with what the body is asking for does take some work, but it's so worth it. And it is the only way that I have seen my clients grow to feel better about their bodies—no matter what their size or shape. How can you take care of something that you loathe?

Start by noticing the times when we are self-critical and apologize to ourselves (literally) for being unkind. We can apologize when it becomes apparent that we've shamed another.

And don't be afraid to respond to family members, doctors, and authority figures when they shame you about weight. Once we accept our bodies (even if we don't love everything about them), then we can start listening to our bodies (Step 4) and stop trying to control or change them. That's when something truly magical happens. We feel lighter within—and connected and whole. We free up our lives for so much more.

Think of the reasons that your friends and loved ones like being around you. If you really can't come up with anything, then boldly ask them. Make a list of the qualities that make you a good friend, sister, partner, parent, employee, pet owner, etc. Maybe it's your ability to make people laugh and feel at ease, the way that you keep a secret, the wonderful hugs that you give. Maybe it's your quiet determination, your strong will, your individuality.

Sandra has a dog that is an extraordinary part of her life. She described how much she loves the dog's body. With keen sensory awareness, she talked about the way the dog feels, his warmth, and the soft pressure as her pooch curls up next to her. It blew Sandra's mind when I replied, "It's *mutual*. The dog loves your body, too!" At first, Sandra looked at me like I had three heads. Then she felt the revelation. This body, the one that she has hated for many decades as she battled anorexia, bulimia, and binge-eating, is actually lovable! In fact, there is a sweet little pup who loves her warmth and softness and cuddliness, and who jumps up and down when he sees her. And this little dog doesn't love just the *idea* of her or who she represents; this little dog loves her *feel*, her *smell*, her actual physical body, just as it is. It was so helpful for my client to see just how relative our feelings about our bodies can be. *The New Oxford American Dictionary* defines *body image* as "the subjective picture or mental image of one's own body." The way that we "see" our bodies can be very different from what others see, especially other beings who love us.

I love being a proud mama and telling the story of my daughter in sixth grade. She told me one day about a group of boys in her class who were judging the girls in the class on how they look. She and her twin sister were in the top three, but she did not like it. To my amazement and delight, she went on to tell me that she marched up to one of the boys and told him to stop this practice. She said, "It makes the girls at the bottom of the list feel bad, and it makes me feel bad, too." What she was trying to articulate is that even being told that you look gorgeous can feel objectifying and wrong. I assured her that she is so much more than a pretty face, and she agreed. I admired her courage and knew that I certainly wouldn't have been so brave in my middle school days.

Make a list of things that you appreciate about yourself. When you feel objectified, or reduced to your looks, or are having one of those "bad body days," then take out this list. Shower yourself with the petals of worth that you wrote down, and remember that you are unique and divine, despite the parts of your body that you'd rather trade in. Take care of that body, and feed it well, as it takes you where you need to go in life; but recognize that it is just one juicy part of the whole that is You. We'll talk more in the next chapter about other strategies when you get stuck in negative body- or self-talk.

Step 2

I want to briefly mention a bit about trauma and the body. Many books have more to say about this topic. I recommend *The Body Keeps the Score,* by Bessel van der Kolk. Sometimes our body loathing and discomfort are related to trauma, such as physical or sexual abuse. When our bodies have been betrayed, we can disconnect from them and distrust them even more. Sometimes when our boundaries have been violated, we try to make ourselves unattractive—consciously or unconsciously—so that it won't happen again. Healing from this trauma and integrating the experience so that we can learn to love and care for our bodies and selves is an important part of the process for some. If your body has been traumatized, healing work that ultimately moves you toward gentleness with yourself will help greatly in this process toward a healthier connection with your body.

That healthy body connection ultimately requires that we let go of the idea that our bodies are bad and need fixing. Then, and only then, can we make choices from a place of self-love, self-respect, and self-care instead of a place of "something's wrong." One of my wise clients shared with me something that she read (author unknown): "What if everyone woke up in the morning and asked, 'How can I bring more love into the world today?' How would our days be different?" At the beginning of this chapter, I quoted Kristin Neff, author of the book *Self-Compassion.* She also wrote, "So why is self-compassion a more effective motivator than self-criticism? *Because its driving force is love, not fear.*" Let's start making our days different by first loving ourselves: Body, mind, and spirit. If you don't really believe you have a lovable body, then spend some time with a dog, as Sandra did. You'll soon see how loved that sweet body of yours can be!

References and Resources

Neff, K. *Self-Compassion: The Proven Power of Being Kind to Yourself.* New York, NY: Harper Collins Publishers, 2011.

Wolf, N. *The Beauty Myth: How Images of Beauty Are Used Against Women.* New York, NY: Harper Collins Publishers, 2002.

Bacon, L. and Aphramor, L. *Body Respect: What Conventional Health Books Get Wrong, Leave Out, and Just Plain Fail to Understand about Weight.* Dallas, TX: BenBella Books, Inc., 2014.

Brown, H. *Body of Truth: How Science, History, and Culture Drive Our Obsession with Weight—And What We Can Do About It.* Boston, MA: Da Capo Press, 2015.

Gaesser, G. *Big Fat Lies: The Truth About Your Weight and Your Health.* Carlsbad, CA: Gurze Books, Inc., 2002.

Van der Kolk, B. *The Body Keeps the Score: Brain, Mind, and Body in the Healing of Trauma.* New York, NY: Penguin Books, 2014.

STEP 3
Awareness Before Action

The more we fear failure, the more frenetically our
bodies and minds work. We fill our days with continual
movement: mental planning and worrying, habitual
talking, fixing, scratching, adjusting, phoning, snacking,
discarding, buying, looking in the mirror. What would
it be like if, right in the midst of this busyness, we were
to consciously take our hands off the controls? What if
we were to intentionally stop our mental computations
and our rushing around and, for a minute or two,
simply pause and notice our inner experience?

~ Tara Brach in *Radical Acceptance*

Do you remember a time when you ate naturally, not thinking about what you were eating or how much of it? Some
of my clients who have had very troubled childhoods might not
be able to remember a time when food—or anything, for that

matter—was simple. Some clients remember a time, before their disordered eating began, when food was easeful. When you watch a toddler eat, you might notice that he will pick up a cookie, enjoy it, and then put it down because something else looks more interesting. That's not something you'll see a lot of adults doing. They'll either avoid the cookies altogether or eat a whole one, not necessarily thinking about how much their bodies want of it. Over time, for many adults, cookies have become a charged food. I'm all for eating for pleasure, but as a little toddler, food was only one of many very exciting and new pleasures. Cookies weren't such a big deal—until their environment turned them into a big deal.

For some individuals, food is significant; for others, it's just not. I believe that some of this is temperamental. My fraternal twin daughters always had different ways with food. Ava is a "foodie" and loved to cook at a young age; she also never missed a snack time and had a hearty appetite, even as a nursing baby. Kyla was a more "picky eater" as a toddler and would rather be doing something else than eating; I would have to remind her that it was time for a meal or snack, otherwise, she would run out of steam. Kyla also used to snooze on and off as an infant during feedings, preferring to nurse a little here and a little there all day. To this day, they have different preferences and styles of eating. It's felt important to me to honor those preferences as I create family meals and pack food for outings. Now that they are preteens, they have more responsibilities around preparing and choosing food in the house, and these responsibilities will increase even more over time. My hope is that they will honor their unique preferences around food and keep listening to their bodies.

Besides temperamental differences around food, there is the environment. I ask very early on in my initial encounter with a client what food was like for her as a child. I love my colleague Christy Harrison's podcast, *Food Psych*. She begins each interview with this same question: "What was your relationship with food like growing up?" Can you remember how you felt about food and eating as a kid? Was it important in your family? Was food scarce at times? Or was it like my client Eleanor described family holidays, where "The table was literally groaning with food"? Did your family express love with food? Was it one of the only ways they showed love? Was food seen as pleasurable or as sinful—or maybe both? Was there a diet culture in your house, where family members were trying to restrict calories or eat clean, such that controlling food was seen as a way of ensuring health, acceptable weight, and wellness?

I encourage you to examine the role that food has played in your life and your family of origin. I find it helpful to my clients to understand where their ideas and patterns with food originated. I also want to foster self-compassion within the person in front of me who feels she has a troubled relationship with food. If she had a charged environment around food all her life, it might reduce self-blame to see the role that environment may have played in her challenges around food. It's not that our families or our culture are *to blame* for our food choices and habits. We all make our own decisions at any given moment. But it is helpful to understand the forces that have encouraged us to make decisions in particular directions. Only with understanding and compassion can we begin to make sustainable changes in these choices. (The key word here is *sustainable*. I do not mean *dieting*.)

Look at your history with food, eating patterns, dieting behaviors, and even various life traumas. This exploration may help you make sense of why food and your body have become a place of conflict. If, after asking yourself questions in this area, you find that your history with food is many layered and complicated, then working with a nutrition therapist and psychotherapist with a specialty in disordered eating can be powerful healing support. I will add that most traditional registered dietitians, psychotherapists, and medical doctors are not trained to work with disordered eating. Uninformed doctors, dietitians, therapists, and psychiatrists can sometimes do more harm than good.

Step 3 is called **Awareness Before Action** for a reason. After two decades of helping people do this work, I finally appreciate that it's difficult to both *notice* what's going on and *change* it at the same time. For example, if Thomas is eating restrictively, this may be setting him up to binge-eat at night. He can't change the evening binge-eating until he notices that he's under-eating the rest of the day, and his nutrition therapist helps to point that out. Thomas learns to appreciate the physiological reason behind the binges: Not eating enough food all day. Thomas also learns over time to understand the psychological/emotional reasons that set him up to binge: Feeling powerless at work, which leaves him frustrated and looking for soothing when he gets home at night. Before he can even change the binge-eating behavior, he increases his awareness of how he's both eating and feeling during the day. I'm not talking about calorie-counting or obsessively monitoring his food, but becoming aware of the fact that he sometimes skips lunch—or feels uncomfortable emotions that bring him to crave pleasure and soothing. If Thomas came into my office saying, "I want to stop binge-eating" and we didn't work on noticing the binge pattern and what leads up to it first, it would be far harder for him to change the behavior.

I often start this process of awareness with some monitoring—but not with a calorie-counting app or Fitbit. (I will admit that I hate those things and find that these devices take us even further out of our bodies, which is the opposite of finding a natural, healthy rhythm with eating and exercise.) I sometimes use a food/feelings journal or diary card from **Dialectic Behavior Therapy® (DBT®)**. Throughout the day, I ask clients to jot down the food they eat, without getting stressed about portions, amounts, or calories counted. Also, they stop to check in before they eat and jot down their thoughts and feelings, as well as a hunger score from zero to ten. (More on that later.) After they eat, they again jot down their thoughts, feelings, and hunger level. Depending on their needs, I might ask them to record physical activity, as well as risks taken or self-care behaviors. Lastly, there is a line for "Today I feel good about _____" to end the self-monitoring on a positive note.

Table 1: Food and Feelings Journal

Food and Feelings Journal   Today's Date: _____

| Time | Before | | Foods & Fluids | Corresponding Events | After | |
	Hunger Level	Thoughts & Feelings			Hunger Level	Thoughts & Feelings

Body Movement

Activity	Length of Time	Thoughts & Feelings	
		Before	After

Risks Taken: _____

Self-Care: _____

Today I feel good about: _____

Heidi Schauster, MS, RDN, CEDRD-S
www.anourishingword.com

I am always amazed at the rich information I get from this exercise. I don't encourage everyone to monitor. Some of my clients have anorexia nervosa or **orthorexia,** a newer term for when obsession with healthy eating takes over one's life. These individuals are already so rigid and obsessed with food and health that recording can intensify the obsessing. If you are already evaluating your food choices so much, it isn't always helpful to do more. For the most part, even for a few days, this exercise may be useful. Try it yourself. What do you notice about your current food habits? Are you mindlessly eating all afternoon, or forgetting to eat until you are starving, or going long stretches without food? Do you eat the same things every day? Do you say negative things to yourself after eating? Do you use "should" and "shouldn't" a lot when you think about food?

What do you notice about your relationship with food as you go through your days?

You will be tempted to try to change some of the behaviors that you don't like right away. Please resist the temptation to do something fast, which is our inclination, especially in today's rapid-paced culture. Instead, just notice what is there without trying to change it. I ask my clients to operate as if they were an investigative reporter and not a critic. Try to suspend judgment, and just take in the facts about your thoughts around food. Also, notice your feelings, but don't judge them as good or bad. Notice the behaviors, and be curious about them. Say, "Hmmmm ... I wonder why I'm always overeating when I have lunch with this friend," instead of, "I'm such an idiot for overeating again." It can take time and practice, but I see this curiosity as a crucial and ongoing part of the process. **Practicing curiosity over judgment and criticism is the most important part of Step 3.** And it continues throughout all of the remaining steps of this process.

So, what do we do when we notice that we are often judging our eating behaviors or ourselves, and we want to become more curious? My favorite exercise that works here is something called **thought defusion** from **Acceptance and Commitment Therapy (ACT)**. I've used this myself and with countless clients with real success. Thought defusion exercises help keep us from getting "hooked" by our thoughts. When we see our thoughts are just words in our heads—and not reality—we have more choice. Of course, it works only if you practice it, and not just once per day. With conscious, daily, regular attention to thoughts and feelings, we may become more skilled at defusion over time.

The thought-defusion exercise that helps the most people I work with is what I call the "I'm having the thought" exercise. (There are many defusion exercises. See Russ Harris's book *The Happiness Trap* for a detailed description of ACT and practical applications.) The gist of the exercise is this. First, you must notice when you have a negative thought. The thought could be about what you are eating or your body, for example. When you have that thought, you might notice that you can give it words, like "I can't believe I ate that ice cream. I shouldn't have done that. I'm such a fat pig." Notice that these (or any other negative thoughts that resonate with you) are words swimming around in your head. They are not facts or "The Truth," but rather a judgment or story that you have in your head about ice cream being bad and your body being wrong. (If it helps, think of another person who might be thinking, "I'm so glad I had that ice cream on a sunny day. It tasted so good, and I feel refreshed. It's so fun to do this with friends.")

The way to put a little distance between your judgment or story and yourself is to change the words in your head around that thought. Instead of saying, "I shouldn't have eaten that ice cream" and "I'm a fat pig," say, "I'm having the thought that I shouldn't have eaten that ice cream. I'm also having the thought that I'm a fat pig." I know it seems a little silly; it's just words. But so are those negative thoughts that have so much power in the first place! You can even take it one step further and say, "I'm noticing that I'm having the thought that I shouldn't have eaten that ice cream. I'm noticing that I'm having the thought that I'm a fat pig." Do you see how you might feel just a little more removed from the idea when you phrase it like this? Instead of being a fat pig, you are just noticing that you are having that thought. If you slow down your mind enough to do this exercise several times a day, you expand around those negative thoughts, see them for what they are, and can decide what to do with them. It's not so easy to know what to do if you are really sinking into being a fat pig. The result is berating yourself or perhaps feeling the need to diet, purge, or exercise the ice cream away, which is ultimately counterproductive to healing your relationship with food and body. If you are only *noticing* you are *having a thought* that you are a fat pig, you can ask yourself what it feels like to have that thought. You can see that these thoughts are demeaning and find something else to occupy your mind. You can do something kind for yourself because you are having these negative body thoughts today and need a little more love and care.

The same is true with feelings. "I notice that I'm feeling anxious and exhausted today" is very different from "I'm anxious and exhausted!" You still have your feelings, but you are noticing them in a way that allows you to pause and perhaps do something to take care of yourself and those feelings. You can be *responsive* instead of being *reactive*. You notice that they are just feelings and that they will run their course, and you can choose how you handle them. Instead of reaching for food when you aren't hungry, for example, which could be a habit when you are on automatic pilot, you can find something else that soothes your anxiety without negative consequences. You might try calling a friend to chat or sitting quietly in a cozy chair and breathing deeply or listening to some soothing music. You may find what floats your boat and helps you manage the anxiety and exhaustion better. **We have to notice that we are anxious and exhausted in the first place. We have more choices when we are using our "observing mind." It's the difference between having feelings and your feelings having you.**

Here's another use of thought defusion that helps compulsive overeaters. After an overeating episode, try saying, "Thank you, Mind. I hear that old story that I screwed up. Instead of being critical of myself, I will look at what happened. I don't feel good right now about how I ate. Why was it that I overate? Maybe I can understand this better so that it is less likely to happen again. What can I do to take care of myself and prevent this from going on in the future?" or "Thank you, Mind. I hear you, but I'm choosing to be curious instead of harsh to myself right now." It may feel alarmingly foreign, but I promise that, if you practice it regularly, you will change your default so that you turn less to criticism and self-flagellation. Instead, you will be more compassionate toward yourself, curious about your eating behaviors, and more prepared for making real changes. Even if you don't believe what you are saying at first—even if you feel that you don't deserve a more compassionate stance—try it. **You deserve to use the kind voice in your mind that you would use when you give a friend or loved one the benefit**

of the doubt. We are all human and imperfect and deserving at our cores. Create the intention to *learn* from your stumbles instead of *becoming* them.

I always say that we can't control the thoughts and feelings that arise in us, though we can learn to respond to them differently when they show up. Thoughts and feelings come and go like clouds in the sky. We can be like the sky, constant and watchful of the cloud passage. What we do have control or choice over are our actions and behaviors—what we do with our limbs, our mouths, our bodies. **When we notice a negative body thought, for example, we can choose to skip a meal to make us feel better (which often backfires into overeating later), or we can investigate our negative body thought and wonder why what we look like today is bothering us so much.** We can then choose to wear more comfortable clothes and, in time, talk to a friend about why we're feeling less than stellar today and get some support.

We can also simply notice that we're having these negative thoughts about our bodies, see that they aren't helpful, and move on to something else. We don't always have to "do" something about negative thoughts. The clouds appear at times, on even the sunniest days. Jon Kabat-Zinn, PhD, meditation teacher, author, and founder of the Stress Reduction Clinic at the University of Massachusetts Medical School, describes mindfulness as learning to surf. Our thoughts and feelings are the waves. We can't stop them, but we can become more skilled at surfing them.

In Step 3, Awareness Before Action, you notice your eating behaviors and patterns even before you decide what you want to change. This process is different from starting with the outcome (for example, weight loss) and then setting goals. This awareness-and-observation period is crucial. Noticing your behaviors around food, eating patterns, feelings and thoughts when you eat, and feelings and thoughts after you eat are all important parts of Step 3. Another bit of noticing comes from digging a little deeper when you find that your eating patterns don't connect with your goals and values. For example, you have a value around self-care, and you want to eat a balanced, health-giving diet, but you find yourself eating foods that ultimately don't make your body feel well. Of course, this requires some listening to your body, which we will talk about more in depth in Step 4. But it also means that we apply that non-judgmental curiosity to those times when our behaviors don't seem to connect with the person we want to be.

Something else is probably up when you find yourself mindlessly eating when you aren't physically hungry, or continuing to eat when you are very full and eating no longer feels right, or restricting food and choosing not to eat when you are indeed hungry. In those moments of disconnect with the body's needs and wants, it is a significant act in this process to stop and ask the question, "What's eating me right now?" Why are you emotionally eating—or restricting and thinking non-stop about food—when you'd rather be spending time with your kids or connecting with a friend or playing in your garden or saving the world?

Why is food getting your attention right now instead of what's really going on? **Sometimes what's really going on is too painful or difficult to deal with, so putting our energy**

into food and our bodies is much easier. If you turn to food, you may do so for excellent reasons. For some people, a full-blown eating disorder can be a lifesaver. Binge-eating or restricting food are coping strategies that work—until they don't anymore and you can see them as having their own unique brand of self-destruction.

Psychological addiction to food or dieting or "perfect" eating can develop. We feel bad; we go to food (indulging or withholding) to soothe these unpleasant feelings. Afterwards, we feel better. The dopamine reward system in the brain gets activated—much less so than our brains on crack or alcohol, but still activated. We learn over time, often unconsciously, that food (or the feeling of denial) is a reward, a treat, something to do when we have feelings that are hard, and we just don't want to deal with them. Unfortunately, as any good therapist or self-help book will tell you, burying feelings just makes them come back all the more strongly at the next appropriate juncture. Not feeling those painful emotions (sadness, anger, grief, disappointment, to name a few) may lead to health problems and difficulties in our relationships.

Noticing the times when we use certain food behaviors (restricting, overeating, binge-eating, purging) to manage painful emotions is critical. Only then can we begin to change the behaviors that we don't like. We need to do something with all those feelings underneath. We can't go around those feelings of grief and loneliness and anger; we need to go through them. I'm always happier when my clients work with a psychotherapist who coordinates the care along with me. While we are changing food behaviors, we often begin to express more emotions and may put new coping strategies into place. If we've been stuffing down feelings with chocolate, for that behavior to change, we need to find new ways of expressing the pain. If we've been starving ourselves and we start to eat again, all that pain underneath can bubble and come to the surface. It's important and so very healing to recognize and move through grief, sadness, anger, and loss; but it sure helps to have support and safe places to express those feelings.

Often we discover that anger and sadness are not so bad. We don't have to eat or starve to deal with our emotions. However, we do need to get used to feeling painful feelings and noticing challenging thoughts. Furthermore, sometimes painful feelings are so familiar that we think it's just the way it's going to be. We loop back to sadness, fear, longing, anger repetitively because these feelings had not been met with openness or kindness before. Meeting our painful feelings with compassion and acceptance—instead of pushing them away may be a new paradigm, but it can be freeing when practiced.

Tara Brach, one of my favorite Buddhist teachers, produced a podcast in April 2017 on Soul Hunger. She so eloquently spoke about how we may have cravings when we are hungry for something else, usually love and attention. We may try to bolster our self-worth through endless achievements, losing x amount of pounds, or eating clean and perfect. Or we might elicit care from others by rendering ourselves chronically sick and exhausted. When we do these things, we lose the present moment, in which we are infinitely worthy and don't need to strive for a sense of value. Instead, when we feel a lack of love and attention, we can turn to ourselves and provide unconditional love and acceptance. If not, we can work with a therapist or healer who can give us that nonjudgmental space until we can accept it ourselves. If we have others in our lives who can provide unconditional love and acceptance, then this is amazing and healing; but we can't rely on others to be there for us at all times. Those wonderful others in our lives have needs, too. So, ultimately, we must find this unconditional love for ourselves. It takes time, if we are used to beating ourselves up, but it's so very worth it. In fact, I believe this self-love is really at the core of having a healthy relationship with food and with our bodies.

What if we've examined our eating patterns, our thought patterns, and our feelings, and we still can't imagine changing them because we've had them since childhood? If you were deprived emotionally as a child and learned to bury feelings to survive, how can you begin to allow yourself to feel some anger and sadness? If you were told over and over by your family and culture that eating less is always better, then how can you accept fullness and find it pleasurable again? There is a fascinating and relatively new understanding that we can change the neural pathways in our brains. Repetitive, unhelpful ways of thinking and being in the world shift when we consciously work to modify the fabric of our minds. Traumatic events may shake us and change our brains in profound ways, particularly when our young brains are forming. But through contemplative practice and techniques that target our unhelpful modes of thinking, we can literally change the way our brains are wired. Science has confirmed it, too, for those who might be skeptical and need more proof.

When we're feeling stuck—when we want to change but seem to find ourselves falling into the same destructive patterns—it's comforting to know that we truly are in charge. We can move toward significant change if we have the right tools. With small acts daily, we build new neural structures in the brain that lead to larger changes as time goes on. The term for this brain changeability is **neuroplasticity**, which means that our brains are really like melty, moldable plastic. I love what one of my group members said one day. She said that everyone else's brain is plastic, but hers is titanium. Everyone laughed and agreed that it's hard to imagine change when we feel stuck, shuffling our feet back and forth over the same grooved path of self-destruction. I have found, however, that the techniques of Acceptance and Commitment Therapy (ACT), and specifically the practice of mindfulness, create profound change and encourage us to move down the road less traveled toward health and well-being.

For example, you need to be *way* slowed down even to use the "I'm having the thought" technique that I mentioned earlier in this chapter. Way ... slowed ... down. If you can do this, you will find that there is something about saying, "Thank you for the teaching moment" that feels much more supportive of change than saying, "Yup, you screwed up again." And how many times do we choose the latter way of talking to ourselves rather than the former?

Okay. Full disclosure. It has taken me a while to sit down and write the pages of this book. I find all kinds of things to distract me. I was doing the self-flagellating thing at first. *There you go, Heidi, procrastinating again. You are lazy, out-of-focus.* I even tried to blame all the people who were interrupting me by phone and email. All of this was not helpful and did not encourage me to write. Then I stopped, observed my mental chatter, and said, "Thank you, Mind. These are old stories and justifications that aren't helping me do what I really want to do. I see them." Slowing down and taking care of myself in a few targeted ways really helped. I acknowledged that I had some unfinished business that I really wanted to attend to first, to feel clear and ready to write. I also had to allow myself the break that my mind needed after seeing clients and before writing. I stopped working altogether for a bit and made a cup of tea for myself. Once I slowed down, listened inside, got clear on what I really wanted to do, and acknowledged the resistance to writing, it became much easier to sit down and begin. I wasn't beating myself up anymore—or trying to flee from that beating by busying myself in another way. When my mind stayed open to what was really going on and got rid of that old story that I was just a procrastinator, lazy, unfocused, well, then, the words flowed.

You are not an idiot who will stay stuck as a binge-eater forever and be powerless in the face of sugar. You are not a former anorexic who is always going to have a funky relationship with food. Stop saying that to yourself (or insert another familiar negative story about your eating or your body). Thank your mind for making the story so clear, and work on creating a new story that is more helpful and supportive of change. Get help with this, if you need to, from a therapist or even from a trusted friend. It can be hard to create new stories when the old ones are so potent. But I do believe, with all my heart—and I've seen this over and over in my practice, as well as in my own life—that you really can change your thoughts and habitual patterns. We now know, by looking at the amazing technology of brain activity, that our brains are, indeed, malleable. We have scientific evidence that, with thought defusion, mindfulness, and meditation, you can change your mind and change your habitual patterns. I'll discuss mindfulness and meditation in more depth soon in Step 4. In my view, the most exciting part about all of this is that, with regular practice, you can ultimately change the course of your life.

References and Resources

Linehan, M. *DBT® Skills Training Manual*. New York, NY: The Guilford Press, 2015.

Harris, R. *The Happiness Trap: How to Stop Struggling and Start Living: A Guide to ACT*. Boston, MA: Trumpeter Books, 2008.

Hayes, S. and Strosahl, K.D. *Acceptance and Commitment Therapy, 2nd Edition: The Process and Practice of Mindful Change*. New York, NY: The Guilford Press, 2016.

Kabat-Zinn, J. *Wherever You Go, There You Are: Mindfulness Meditation in Everyday Life*. New York, NY: Hachette Books, 2005.

Podcast: Christy Harrison's *Food Psych*

STEP 4

Body Trust and
Deep Listening

If we allow ourselves to align with and listen to our feelings
and our bodies, we can use them as our guides. If we listen
and attune to our bodies and our feelings, they can help us
make decisions that support our growth. They can be our
antennae, moving us away from that which causes pain,
harm, and disconnection in our lives and toward people,
places, and opportunities that meet our innermost needs.

~ Sondra Kronberg, MS, RDN, CEDRD

I f you've moved with me through the last few Steps, you've
been trying to ditch the diet mentality, accept your unique
body, and build some awareness about the eating patterns that
you wish to change. There is much work to be done before we
take action to change any habit. Step 4 takes the Awareness
process in Step 3 further. I call this Step **Body Trust and Deep**

Listening because it involves developing a deeper connection with your body so that you can use that connection to make choices around food, exercise, sleep, and other practices and habits that resonate with who you are. Body trust and deep listening encourage care for your body and being.

There are lots of ways to connect with our bodies. Conscious movement is one way, and I'll cover physical activity and exercise later in much more detail. Most movement, dance, and yoga therapists would agree that we have greater access to feelings and healing when we move than if we just talk or use our mind. Motion and non-verbal work can bring about shifts in the body/mind/spirit in very profound ways. In a discussion of body trust, it's worth mentioning movement and exercise, but it's such an important topic that I made it into Step 6. We'll visit it soon.

If someone is suffering from **anorexia nervosa** and has been eating restrictively for some time, the body's signals and communication may be difficult to read. Step 4, Body Trust and Deep Listening, may not be possible in these individuals without significant treatment to restore weight and nutritional status first. That said, many who struggle with restriction of food can do this step once they are in less medical danger and their brains are better fed. The body-mind connection works poorly in severe starvation.

On the most basic level, if you wish to cultivate deep listening and body trust, you must first slow down. I mean s.l.o.w. … d.o.w.n. … We are not typically encouraged to do this in our fast-paced do-it-all-and-then-do-more culture. Based on my personal and clinical experience, I firmly believe that you will struggle to make change happen in your life (on all fronts, not just in your eating patterns) if you don't slow down, listen deeply, and trust your body. Presence in our bodies and our lives brings consciousness, and consciousness creates the space for change.

If we don't take the time to listen and actually hear what our bodies are trying to tell us—hunger, fullness, pain, tiredness, restlessness, cravings, nervous flutterings, other sensations—we miss out on a form of communication from which we might learn so much. This communication truly helps us to make decisions that bring us to live more abundant, full, and meaningful lives. Through our bodies, we get in touch with our deepest needs and feelings. When we have that connection and awareness to our needs and feelings, then we are better able to meet them. When our needs are more readily met, then we have a stronger chance of being able to help and support other people we care about as well.

It's rather trite, but I'm going to say it anyway. We can't help a child in a plane emergency if our own oxygen mask is not in place first. If we are gasping for air and not taking care of ourselves, those we care about on this path we call living will suffer, too. I used to believe that being a martyr and serving all above myself was the road to enlightenment. **I've learned the hard way (and so have many of my clients) that the most loving act you can offer those you care about is to love, respect, and care for yourself first. In doing so, you bring freedom and spaciousness for connection, compassion, and the blossoming of deeper, more caring relationships.** This self-care takes practice if you weren't trained this way from a young age, but it's possible to learn. You will transform yourself and your relationships in the process. I believe that we need to use our minds to grow and change, but we also need to listen to the wisdom of our bodies and the feelings housed in our bodies—particularly if we want to find a more easeful, nourishing relationship with food and eating.

I love this segment about compulsive eating from an article by Geneen Roth that I posted on my blog, with her permission, in 2013.

Most of us secretly believe that good people, especially women, take care of others first. They wait until everyone else has a plateful and then take what's left. Unfortunately, most of us make decisions based on our ideas of who we think we should be, not on who we are. The problem is, when we make choices based on an ideal image of ourselves—what a good friend would do, what a good mother would do, what a good wife would do—we end up having to take care of ourselves in another way.

Enter food. When you don't consider your real needs, you will likely fill the leftover emotional hunger with food. (Or another abused substance. Or shopping. But most of us opt for food.) You eat in secret. You eat treats whenever you can because food is the one way, the only way, you nourish yourself. You eat on the run because you believe that you shouldn't take time for lunch; there's too much work to do. You eat the éclair, the doughnut, the cake, all the while knowing this isn't really taking care of yourself. But to take care of yourself, you have to think of yourself first.

I believe that compulsive overeating, restrictive eating, or eating obsessively "clean" can be a way to reward and take care of a self that you repeatedly put last. So, how do we begin to take better care of ourselves, learn how to get in touch with the body's wisdom, and s.l.o.w. d.o.w.n.? First, I must put in a plug for meditation practice. There are many ways to meditate, and there are countless books and audio files on meditation. (I list some of my favorites at the end of this chapter.) I have taken courses, listened to recordings, and tried many different forms of meditation, and I encourage you to explore what works for you. Personally, I made meditation a daily practice (and, therefore, found the profound benefits of it) only when I committed to practicing ten minutes of insight-oriented meditation every day. I had to let go of needing to do it for longer. I had to let go of doing it every morning. I stayed with it only if I committed to doing it every day and could fit it in whenever my day allowed it. I also had to let go of the resistance that I had to meditate and realize that the resistance is also a piece of learning. I had to let go of the part of me that wanted to do it perfectly and find a way to accept my distracted monkey mind. Sometimes I allow myself more stillness and reflection than ten minutes, but I allow myself a practice of pure presence every day. I finally got to a point where I decided that I deserved ten minutes just to *be* (and not *do*) every day. If I couldn't cultivate that, then how could I teach others to listen deeply and be present?

Once I made that daily commitment to meditation, I could not believe the results. Of course, I had heard everything about it being relaxing—creating more calmness and less anxiety—which sounded great. I had no idea that it would improve my life in so many other ways. I felt like a fog was slowly lifting. I could see more clearly during so many moments each day. I became more in touch with myself, my decisions were easier, my self-doubt decreased, and I stood up for myself more. I felt more compassion for my shortcomings and was able to work on them with humility. I was even more loving and present for my family and friends.

Now, mind you, everything isn't always hunky-dory. In some ways, meditation practice has allowed me to feel more of life's fullness, which means the downs as well as the ups. When I'm sad about something, I get more in touch with that in the quiet space on my cushion. When I'm angry, I feel that come up and, as a result, may choose to confront the person involved. That part's not so fun. I'm more in touch with my feelings, so I express them more. Some people in my life welcome that, and sometimes it creates waves. If the other person is also aiming to be honest and present, that can occasionally be messy. Sometimes it's beautiful, vulnerable, and connective, and we arrive at a deeper, more respectful place. Sometimes it's just messy. But I know that my own meditation practice has helped me with something I call **discernment**: A stronger understanding and clearer ability to make decisions about others and my surroundings. And it's also helped me to be far more present in my life and relationships.

Now I'll get to the reason you are reading this book. Meditation practice also forces me to get in touch with my body. I notice if I feel tired or fatigued, or if there is a twinge in my leg that is telling me to be gentle when I'm dancing later in the day. I notice if there is anxiety because I feel it in my head and chest. I notice if my heart feels heavy. I notice if my body feels light and energized and how that's different from the day before. I don't judge or ascribe meaning to these changes. My mind mightily tries to, but I try to gently thank my mind for its concern and move back to my body and to clear presence. I have to do this over and over and over again. I notice that, when I'm tired, I have to do it more. I notice that, when I'm exhausted, I can barely find that quiet, present place. (No wonder I don't relate to my family the way I want to when I'm exhausted!)

Sometimes a quiet, meditative walk (without music or my phone, just noticing what there is to notice and being in the present moment and not in my head) has the same quality. In fact, I find that I can do almost any task in the spirit of presence and that doing so is indeed nourishing, even if it is not quite the same thing as my daily meditation practice. There is a place for planning and organizing (I couldn't have written this book without it). However, getting out of our heads and into our bodies and senses is an important part of the process of healing our relationships with food. Presence also gives us respite from our noisy lives. Although I've reaped much deeper rewards from a daily stillness meditation, I also have learned that my body needs movement and find that meditative moving can be very beneficial. Moving or walking meditation may create less resistance for some over traditional, seated meditation. It can certainly be a place to start.

So why am I singing the praises of meditation in a book about healing your relationship with food and body? Because I believe that meditation is a path to connect with the body— and soul—and I will admit that it took me years (years!) to find a way to meditate that actually worked with my being and lifestyle. Then, it took me some time to get comfortable with it. In fact, I go through waves when I'm more distracted and uncomfortable with meditation even now. I learn a lot from that discomfort. It usually means I'm afraid of what might come up in that stillness. I honestly don't want you to waste another day without the incredible transformative power of this practice. And I believe that the benefits are subtle at first, until you get comfortable with the process. Again, a meditation coach, book, or video can be invaluable. Think about how you learn best and find your own way.

So, what if you hate your body so much that the idea of getting more in touch with it is terrifying or uncomfortable? One of my clients shared with me that, in meditation and in physical exercise (she's beginning to practice both), she notices how uncomfortable she feels with the fat on her body. Another client who wishes to gain weight gets in touch with how weak her muscles feel and how sore her body feels just sitting still. Both of these women feel lousy when they get in touch with their bodies. As difficult as these feelings are, they are important body messages. As I discussed in Step 2, we are invited to respond to these feelings with compassion and acceptance. Only then, from a place of nonjudgmental, kind regard, can we decide how best to care for our bodies as they are.

Sustainable change sprouts from compassion and not loathing. I have seen this over and over and over again in more than two decades of practice, and I just can't say it enough. If you don't feel that you can deeply listen to and find acceptance with your body, I would recommend going back to Step 2 and spending more time there. It's an area that often requires some work. Find a body-positive, Health-At-Every-Size (HAES) psychotherapist, nutrition therapist, or coach if you need some help and support here.

What does Body Trust entail? If you are reading this book, chances are you aren't trusting your body's signals much. Somewhere along the line, you might have stopped listening to the wisdom of your body that says things like, "I'm really in the mood for soup," "I feel like I need some heavier, grounding food," or "I have a real taste for squash but not tomatoes." Sometimes our bodies crave unusual foods, like the pregnant semi-vegetarian woman who suddenly wants to eat meat much more often. (This is not uncommon when she needs extra protein and iron to grow a baby.) Sometimes our bodies want to eat more food when we have been more active, especially if we are using new muscles. Women usually require more food toward the end of their menstrual cycles, when metabolism increases; hence, premenstrual cravings. Ever wonder why you suddenly feel like you want to eat some fish? Or why a sandwich is more appealing than a salad some days but not others? Our bodies have lots of wisdom about what we need; we just have to listen.

Setting up foods as "good" or "bad"—or always choosing the "healthy" or "low-calorie" option—overrides the body's good judgment about what to eat. Maybe you are out of practice with actually listening to your body. Perhaps you aren't used to listening to hunger and don't even know what your real food preferences are these days. For example, you might think you like a particular food, but you aren't sure that you feel terrific after eating it.

Evelyn Tribole and Elyse Resch are the gurus of **Intuitive Eating**. In 1995, I read their new book and was blown away. Fortunately, I started my nutrition career at this time and under the influence of this book. When Tribole and Resch began their careers, they were registered dietitians doing weight-loss counseling. They noticed it wasn't working and organically came up with a paradigm that did not include the dieting they had been instructing clients to do for years. They began to promote listening to hunger and fullness, coping with emotions without using food, and what they called "gentle nutrition" to honor health and well-being. Intuitive Eating is woven into my 10 Steps because it was the foundation of my nutrition practice, as well as a part of my healing from an eating disorder. I've encouraged the majority of my clients to read *Intuitive Eating* if they haven't already. I'm encouraging you in Step 4 to embrace deep listening and body trust. This confidence in your body takes both intuitive eating and mindfulness practice and blends them, so that food-behavior change (Step 5) is possible.

I am aware that I'm repeating myself here, but, this time, my suggestion is to s...l...o...w... d...o...w...n... the process of eating. Mindful eating is slow, and many of us rarely eat this way. (I mindlessly eat lunch while I check email more than I'd like to admit.) Try to eat slowly and deliberately sometime when you are alone and undistracted. It could be a challenge! Mindfulness is a bit of a buzzword these days. The dictionary defines **mindfulness** as "the quality or state of being conscious or aware of something" or "a mental state achieved by focusing one's awareness on the present moment, while calmly acknowledging and accepting one's feelings, thoughts, and bodily sensations, used as a therapeutic technique."

In short, mindfulness is a practice of paying full, non-judgmental attention to our moment-to-moment experience. It sounds rather simple, but, in practice, mindfulness can be challenging—particularly in our fast-paced, multi-tasking world. When you begin to cultivate mindfulness in your eating experiences, amazing things happen (but not overnight). Gradually, and with practice, I have witnessed many chaotic, disconnected eaters begin to identify the triggers to their food choices and behaviors. They also begin to question whether those choices and behaviors are in their best interest and start to make choices that are more aligned with health (if they are, indeed, interested in health) and self-care.

One of my favorite mindfulness techniques is what I call "the Zen of chopping vegetables." I use this particularly with clients who overeat compulsively, but anyone who occasionally eats mindlessly could benefit. You don't have to do it with vegetables. The exercise is all about taking in the sensory environment of whatever foods you prepare. It's just that veggies are so colorful and make such a satisfying sound when cut. (So much so that, when I cut something on a wooden cutting board, the sound would make our family's pet guinea pigs in the other room squeak in Pavlovian excitement.)

I'm sure you have chopped vegetables. But have you *actually* chopped vegetables? I'm talking about clearing the clutter from your heads, examining that juicy carrot in its fullness of color and crispness, and then cutting away. Notice the sound, the texture, the rhythm of the knife on the cutting board. Now take a vegetable of a different color and texture. Hear the different sound the blade makes on the board, the change in juiciness, the feel of the experience. Notice the patterns on the inside of the vegetable. This exercise may be exposing the secret that prep chefs in restaurant kitchens know already: Preparing food can be relaxing, transporting, sensual.

When you get bored of being so in tune with what you are doing (and you will—it's the nature of the mind), then imagine where the food comes from, who grew it, who tended it, and how it got to your kitchen—all the many steps. Acknowledge the miracle that is our nourishment. Now, chop some more. Tune in to the other parts of the meal with the same mindful attention, as if this was going to be your last meal and you want to savor the experience and life in it. You may notice that the process of preparing food can be almost as nourishing as eating it. Almost.

Now, I hear you say, "When in the world do I have time to chop vegetables like this? I only have a half hour to get dinner on the table for a family of four!" I hear you. Most of the time, I can't Zen-out in the kitchen, either. But, I guarantee that if you commit to mindful food-preparation practice at least once per week (and ideally more in small doses here and there), you will enjoy those less-mindful kitchen times more. You will have slowly but surely re-wired your brain to relax and nourish yourself more in the act of feeding yourself and others. Instead of a "should" or a "chore," food preparation can feel like taking good care of your body and soul. It can be a peaceful respite from life's more stressful thoughts, feelings, and activities.

Again, this won't happen overnight. But by cultivating awareness, nonjudgmental attention, and gratitude for the foods that you are preparing, you will slowly appreciate the act of feeding yourself differently. There is little room for obsession, judgment, and mindless binge-eating in the purest form of this sort of practice. If you notice judgment, emotions, or thoughts come up, do notice them. Then, return your focus to self-care, gratitude, and the sounds and smells that are before you. Right now. Try mindful food preparation and see what it does for your eating and self-care. It's just one of many mindfulness practices that clients have found helpful on the path toward balanced, self- and body-attuned eating. The act of taking food preparation slowly—the way we used to do it out of necessity—can be healing, relaxing, and sometimes meditative. But you want to allow yourself space and know that it won't be easy at first. The simple act of preparing a colorful vegetable or fruit salad—or any baked good or main dish, for that matter—actually can be nourishing on so many sensory levels. Allow yourself the time and attention and spaciousness to notice.

Then, take that mindfulness into your actual eating experiences. I encourage you to pause before you prepare a meal (if you have the choice) and ask yourself what you want to eat. What textures, flavors, and temperatures would be appealing? Try not to let your ideas about health or nutrition dictate your choices. You may have to get quiet and still to read your body's signals.

Other ways to slow down and eat more mindfully include taking in the visual appeal of the food and the smell before even taking a bite. Make this a sensual experience! Then, I invite you to ask yourself how hungry you are for this food. Is it stomach hunger, or is your mouth or nose or mind hungry for it mainly? Some people find it helpful to rate their hunger on a scale of 1 to 10, considering their mouth hunger, nose hunger, eye hunger, stomach hunger, and whole body hunger separately. I first tried this exercise at a conference in a workshop with Jan Chozen Bays, author of *Mindful Eating*. I am always surprised at how different the numbers are when I do this exercise with clients. Sometimes we think we need to eat, but our senses just want a break from the computer screen, even while our bodies and stomachs are quite satisfied or full.

Some of my clients say they benefit from thinking about where the food came from right before they eat—all the people, animals, plants, sunshine, and rain that made the meal possible. They try to feel real gratitude for the food instead of wolfing it down fast. Doing so creates a reverence and respect for the process of eating, and they slow down more naturally, finding it easier to listen to their bodies when they are eating more mindfully.

When I'm doing a mindful-eating exercise with a client, I encourage him to take a few slow bites and notice the flavor, texture, and feel of the food in his mouth. I encourage him to savor the pleasure of eating each bite. For some of my clients, especially those who have sexual-abuse histories or upbringings that stressed a denial of pleasure, this can be difficult. Experiencing the sensual pleasure of eating can feel wrong on some level—conscious or unconscious—and may contribute to "tuning out" when eating. **If you notice yourself tuning out and moving out of a full-bodied experience of eating, then gently invite yourself back to the table.** Stay with the sensations of eating as much as you can. This practice is harder to do if you are eating with others or if you are distracted by your surroundings (or email). I invite you to choose a few mindful meals per week and see what happens. If you like the results, you can eat more meals and snacks like this.

An essential part of the mindful-eating process—particularly as I see it in healing our relationships with food and body—is to get in touch with those vital sensations of hunger and fullness. Try asking yourself where your body is on a scale of 0 to 10—where 0 is the most hungry you can imagine, and 10 is the most full you can imagine. You might start by closing your eyes right now and asking that question. If you have trouble getting in touch with your sensations of hunger and fullness, then it's worth practicing this many times per day—before, during, and after meals. I occasionally recommend that clients set an alert on their phones to go off at random times per day. When they hear the signal, they are invited to get in touch with their hunger/fullness and give it a rating. It's also a good time to check in around any feelings that might be present, too. There are a lot of factors that affect appetite; what I hear about most often is that hunger and fullness are often present but tuned out. Here's an example. Think about a time when your hunger level got to a 1 or 2. You were in the middle of a project, completely immersed, and then you finally couldn't ignore your hunger any longer. Under these conditions, most people will overeat (to about an 8 or 9). It's human nature to eat fast and too much when there is a sense of scarcity.

I love the diagram on the next page from the Oliver Pyatt Center, a program that treats eating disorders, including Binge Eating Disorder. I find it especially helpful for those who struggle to feel a connection with their bodies. The second Emotional

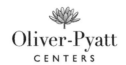

Oliver-Pyatt
CENTERS

Hunger/Fullness *Scale*

physical cues

Appetite and/or cravings can occur

Satiety occurs

4 — SENSE SPACE IN STOMACH

5 — TRANSITIONAL

6 — SENSE FOOD IN STOMACH

3 — HUNGRY

7 — SUBTLE FULLNESS

2 — STRONG HUNGER

8 — FULL

1 — EXTREME HUNGER

9 — EXTREME FULLNESS

0 — EMPTY

10 — PAINFULLY FULL

emotional cues

0	1	2	3	4	5	6	7	8	9	10
COGNITIVE DETERIORATION / NUMB	INABILITY TO FOCUS / HEIGHTENED IRRITABILITY	PREOCCUPIED WITH FOOD / URGENCY TO RESPOND	CLEAR, RECOGNIZABLE CUES / FOOD TASTES GOOD	SLIGHT HINTS OF INTEREST IN FOOD	LACK OF INTEREST IN FOOD	FLEETING THOUGHTS OF FOOD	EMOTIONALLY SATISFIED / EATING IS LESS ENJOYABLE	DECREASED OR NO DESIRE TO CONTINUE EATING	EMOTIONAL AND/OR PHYSICAL DISCOMFORT	PROFOUND, DISTRACTING FULLNESS

Cues diagram often resonates more than the first Physical Cues diagram for these individuals. Some clients can't discern when they feel hungry in their bodies, but they notice when they are feeling spacey, irritable, and "hangry."

When you are practicing a mindful meal, check in with your hunger level before you start to eat. After several slow, enjoyable bites, ask yourself how hungry you still are for this food. Repeat the process every so often, staying connected to the sensations of eating (taste, smell, touch, texture, etc.). Notice when you are getting full. What does that feel like in your body? How do you know when to stop? Notice the sensations. I have heard many different descriptions of hunger and fullness. What do they feel like in your particular body?

If this practice sounds simple to you, that's because it is. Regardless, many of us have lost the ability to eat in this attuned way. Eating with care and nurturance also feeds our souls and hearts. Try it even with a few bites each day. You will see a difference in your relationship with food start to emerge. Many of my clients who practice mindfulness in their eating report that they feel more deeply nourished when they eat this way; they feel cared for. If they are also finding other ways to feed themselves outside of meals, with activities, people, and time to re-energize, then food takes its place as just one of the many pleasures in their lives.

Many of my clients with anorexia nervosa need to restore regular eating and healthy weight gain before they can even begin to tune in to their bodies. Their bodies and minds are starved, confused, and in need of basic nutritional needs first. Sometimes it can be a long process of healing, but it starts with trusting yourself and your body—not the newest diet or the next "Top Ten Perfect Foods" list.

We are all perfectly imperfect. So is our food. Eat what you like. Eat what makes you feel good in each very different moment. Some days it feels good to eat a hearty meal. Sometimes that same meal will feel too heavy and not right. Each time you eat and notice how your body feels, you learn something about what your body likes and doesn't like. You learn about what foods feel good and what foods don't. Food allergies and sensitivities are complicated and hard to identify. There are many books on this topic out there, and everyone has a slightly different take on what it means to be sensitive or allergic to different foods. A registered dietitian/nutrition specialist can help you sort this out, and we'll talk more about this in Step 9. Gastrointestinal (GI) symptoms can also cloud a clear picture of what the body needs. Sometimes these symptoms need treatment before this process can be entirely helpful, and sometimes this process amazingly clears up the GI symptoms.

What I have found in practice, though, is that once clients go through the first 4 Steps and get practiced at recognizing hunger and fullness cues, they are more ready to go on to Step 5. In Step 5, they begin to play around with finding the way of eating that resonates with them and their unique bodies. They start to change their food habits. They discover which foods, food combinations, and eating styles feel good to them and which foods don't. So many who struggle with disordered eating don't get help with this. They flounder for years around food, feeling disconnected and confused about what they should or shouldn't eat. This is where the healing begins. I don't tell my clients what to eat more of or what to eat less of. I might point out some imbalances, given my nutrition-science background. But I'm much more interested in what my clients discover on this journey of listening deeply and trusting the cues and sensations of the body.

If you regularly weigh yourself, I recommend that you decrease—and ideally ditch—the dance with the scale. It's hard to listen to your body's cues around hunger and fullness if you are using the number on the scale to tell you what or how much you should eat. That is an external signal, much like a diet (which I hope you abandoned after Step 1). This 10-step healing process is all about trusting your internal cues about what and how much to eat. Let's say your weight is up a couple of pounds today. The weight gain could be related to hydration, water retention, or the presence of food in the stomach or intestines—as compared to the last time you checked your weight. If you weigh yourself frequently, you know that your weight is lowest in the morning and increases naturally over the course of the day. You also may know that it fluctuates—going up or down in a way that sometimes doesn't seem to have any rhyme or reason when you compare it to your eating patterns. Many of my clients are just astounded by the sense of freedom that ditching the scale provides. Some of them smash it, throw it out windows, or hide it in my office closet until they feel able to let it go. Losing the scale makes most people feel, not ironically, like a tremendous weight was lifted. It's a major stepping stone in the process of trusting our bodies and ourselves to make food decisions based on self-care and not punishment or restraint.

Of course, your doctor may need to monitor your weight because it is too low or because you have a thyroid or other condition that affects your weight. I can't see any other reason to monitor body weight outside of a medical visit or check-up. Most people are aware of shifts in their weight without needing a scale to put a number to it. In fact, some people start an exercise program and get discouraged because their weight initially goes up. Muscle weighs more than fat, so working out may make you leaner without changing weight very much. If you use the scale as your guide when you change your physical activities, you may be underestimating your progress in taking good care of your body. Go back to Step 2 if you need more help with body acceptance. Step 2 is a place that many go back to, as we live in a culture that puts far too much emphasis on weight and less on a healthy connection with our bodies.

I invite you to get quiet, deeply listen, trust your body, and use your internal cues and sense of well-being to help you make decisions about food and other self-care practices. I invite you to be very interested in what your body is telling you when you eat—before, during, and after. Pay careful attention to the wisdom of your very own body. It will serve you well as you move on to Step 5, where taking action to change eating habits and practices begins.

References and Resources

Roth, G. *Women, Food, and God.* New York, NY: Scribner/ Simon and Schuster, 2010.

Kornfield, J. *Meditation for Beginners*. Boulder, CO: Sounds True, Inc., 2008.

Chodron, P. *How to Meditate: A Practical Guide to Making Friends with Your Mind*. Boulder, CO: Sounds True, Inc., 2013.

Chozen Bays, J. *Mindful Eating: A Guide to Rediscovering a Healthy and Joyful Relationship with Food*. Boston, MA: Shambhala Publications, 2009.

Tribole, E. and Resch, E. *Intuitive Eating: A Revolutionary Program That Works*. New York, NY: St. Martin's Press, 2012.

Podcast: Tara Brach

STEP 5

Mindful Eating with Nutritional Common Sense

Because of the media hype and woefully inadequate
information, too many people nowadays are deathly afraid
of their food, and what does fear of food do to the digestive
system? I am sure that an unhappy or suspicious stomach,
constricted and uneasy with worry, cannot digest properly.
And if digestion is poor, the whole body politic suffers.

~ Julia Child (1912–2004)

The health and nutrition fields provide us with so much
contradicting information that it can be hard to know
how to feed ourselves well. One year's health-food hero becomes
another year's health-food monster. (If you are old enough to
remember, margarine was embroiled in this controversy.) **Variety
and moderation are not very sexy. They don't sell diet books
and pills and plans, but they're still the gold standard when**

it comes to food and health. Moderation means that there aren't good and bad foods. It means that food is one form of (self-) love and that all foods can be lovable.

Step 5 is where the action happens. Notice that we have to do some Acceptance, Awareness, Listening, and Trusting before we take Action and make changes in our relationship with food. Don't be alarmed if you struggle with Step 5. It's the step that many of us get stuck at because it requires a fair amount of preparation and hard work. You may have to drop back to Steps 1, 2, 3, or 4 and revisit them when you are feeling stuck. Remember, this process is not designed to be linear. To make changes, we need to have space, time, and energy to invest in those changes. We need to believe in ourselves and be able to go head-to-head with any resistance that comes up. (And, please do count on at least some resistance in this Step!) We need to be gentle with ourselves, understanding that our food habits (no matter how weird) are there for a reason—and perhaps served an important purpose. We have to cultivate real consciousness to change them.

In my practice, once clients are ready and have worked through Steps 1 to 4, we then begin to work on mindful, intuitive, nourishing eating. We investigate habits that feel worth putting the time and attention into to change. **I think many books on nutrition are all wrong. They tell us how to eat and what to eat and when to eat without honoring the body's wisdom.** I am going to talk about nutrition and food here because this is the information that so many seek. As I talk about diet and nutrition, though, I will attempt to remind you to listen deeply to your very own body and preferences. I call this **Mindful Eating with Nutritional Common Sense.** You know that eating a candy bar for dinner doesn't feel right, but how do you decide what to eat instead? A little basic nutritional knowledge can go a long way toward helping you make choices that feel good and support a vital body and mind.

First, a brief review of **mindful eating practices** from Step 4, so that they don't get lost in all the discussion of nutrition and food. The most important principles, as I see them, are:

- **Slowing down and paying attention**

- **Witnessing the thoughts, emotions, and sensations that come up around eating**

- **Being curious, not critical, of your choices and the eating process**

- **Getting to know your hunger and fullness cues**

- **Knowing that you are ultimately the expert on what you like and what your body prefers**

A last mindful-eating practice that will serve you well on this journey is **Eating with Gratitude.** Appreciating the miracle and many steps that brought the food to your table (or desk) for just a moment before eating will not only slow you down and drop you into mindfulness, but it's an antidote for all of the analyzing, counting, obsessing, and questioning that might precede a meal or snack. With your heart full of appreciation and gratitude for the plants, animals, and humans that made your food possible, you are better able to see eating as an act of self-care.

With that overview, I'm going to now discuss nutrition and health and how it figures into this more nourishing, mindful way of approaching your body and food. Remember in the Introduction, when I wrote that I didn't feel that I could recommend a good basic book on nutrition to most of my clients with a clear conscience? In this chapter, I'm trying to provide the basics for you. These are the nutritional concepts that I find myself explaining over and over in my work and the ones that clients tell me are helpful. One of my goals in writing this book has been to create the much-sought-after manual about "How to Eat" that doesn't take away from the inner wisdom in each of us, but still communicates some basic nutritional principles. These principles will ideally help you to feed your body in such a way that provides you with energy, feels good, and allows you to experience eating as an act of self-care on a deep level.

Sometimes we get into habits with food, and we think that they are best for us. "I never eat breakfast" or "I always eat this for lunch, and it works for me," are fine statements; but I encourage you to expand your nutritional horizons, try some different ways of eating, and apply the deep listening of Step 4. Then you can honestly say with conviction that the way you are eating feels kind and care-taking. You may be surprised at what you find when you try on different ways of eating. Sometimes we have to teach the body to eat well because it's so used to not feeling well. It just doesn't know any better.

I'll give you an example. Nicole never ate mid-afternoon between lunch and dinner and said she didn't want or need to do so. "Why would I want to plan to eat more when I'm already unhappy about my tendency to overeat and my weight?!" We scrutinized her eating patterns and noticed a gap of seven hours between lunch and dinner and a tendency to overeat at dinner, which ultimately made her feel lousy physically and emotionally. She did a Food Experiment with me and added a balanced snack mid-afternoon, around 4:00 p.m. At this time, she started to get hungry but would typically ignore the hunger sensation until it went away. Adding the snack was a significant change; she virtually stopped her nightly overeating in its tracks. In the end, she ended up eating less food, more evenly spaced out in her day. Her energy was more stable and consistent. She enjoyed eating dinner more because she was less ravenous and could tune in to the flavors and downtime of the meal. I've shared a simple example, and maybe an obvious one to you; but it was not apparent to Nicole until she played around with something new and realized that it brought her eating more into balance.

When you know a little bit about basic nutrition, anatomy, and physiology, it can be enlightening. (Also in the Introduction, I told you how this helped me in my recovery from restrictive and binge-eating patterns.) Unfortunately, I've also learned that when you know a *lot* about nutrition science, you recognize that it's bound to change completely in the next few years! Nutrition in health and chronic disease is a relatively new, ever-evolving field of study. So, I'm sticking here to the nutritional basics to help you heal your relationship with food. While my bias is always on listening to your body and preferences in any given hungry moment, I find that many people are perplexed about how to eat well for energy, clarity, and vitality. Humans all over the world eat and thrive in many different ways. I do not believe that there is one right way to eat, but cuisines the world over have some basic principles of balance in common that have encouraged their people to thrive. Here are some of those basic principles. These are the nutritional nuggets that my clients have told me, again and again, are helpful to them in creating a rhythm with food that allows them to listen deeply and feed themselves well.

Core Macronutrients: Carbohydrates, Proteins, Fats

Nutrition is not rocket science. It's a bit of biochemistry (which were not my favorite college courses, I'll admit). The biochemistry of eating can be boiled down to the taking in and assimilating of the three primary macronutrients— **Carbohydrates, Proteins, and Fats**—as well as the micronutrients, which include **Vitamins and Minerals**. The macronutrients are our fuel or gasoline. The micronutrients are like the spark plugs of the car; they are essential for our bodies to run well, but not the primary fuel source driving us. Vitamins and minerals help to convert food into energy; heal wounds and damage to cells; boost the immune system; strengthen bones; and produce hormones, blood cells, and neurotransmitters. Carbohydrates get broken down into glucose, proteins into amino acids, and fats into fatty acids. These are the smallest parts and building blocks of most major processes in the body. Without all three of these macronutrients, our diets and bodies are unbalanced, so they are worth some time in our discussion of a healthy relationship with food.

Carbohydrates

I'm going to spend a little more time on this macronutrient, as I think it's the most misunderstood. When Anna eats too few carbohydrates (all too common today with low-carb-diet popularity), she typically feels hungry much of the time, low in energy, and tends toward sugar cravings. Those cravings are the body's way of trying to get more glucose into the body. Carbohydrates are the only energy source for the brain. They are crucial to the rest of your body, too. When athletes "carbo load" at a pasta dinner the night before a big race, they are making sure that plenty of stored carbohydrate is available for the muscles to draw on. If you don't eat enough carbohydrate, your body will take the protein from your muscle, break it down into amino acids, and then convert these to glucose. Athletes don't want that happening. Carbohydrates are found in most foods but primarily in grains, fruits, vegetables, and dairy products. These foods provide readily available energy. At the risk of sounding woo-woo to my more science-oriented friends, I consider carbohydrate-rich foods to be very grounding food. I can often sense when clients are low in carbohydrates. They are scattered, kind of chaotic in their speech and demeanor, and they can't stop thinking about food.

"Aren't we eating too many carbs, though?" many clients ask. "It's not a good idea to eat up the whole breadbasket before eating a meal, right?" Of course not. Moderation, while not a very popular word in the health lexicon, is always advised with eating. In fact, if one tunes in and eats mindfully, moderation is what will keep coming up. The United States public health message that we need to decrease our carbohydrate intake comes from the fact that our muffins are gigantic, our consumption of sugary soda is excessive, and the super-sizing of everything from ice cream cones to sandwiches is significant. Over the last several decades, typical portion sizes of high-carbohydrate foods have increased, and this makes it increasingly hard to eat moderately and trust our instincts. It's hard for us to decide when we are full and have had enough to eat when large portion sizes are commonplace.

That said, restricting carbohydrates is *not* the answer! One of the members of my No Diet Book Clubs once said, "Anytime there is a suggestion of deprivation, I go crazy." As many weight-loss-diet veterans will agree, taking away foods creates a state of deprivation, which often leads to cravings and overeating of the "bad" foods. Overeating commonly shows up when someone significantly decreases their carbohydrate foods—especially grain products, like rice, whole grains (oats, quinoa, millet, etc.), bread, cereals, and pasta. In fact, I find that when someone eats less of these foods per day than their body needs, they often crave sugar, the simplest form of carbohydrate.

When a client complains about frequent binge-eating or overeating at night, there is often an emotional or stress-related trigger. But, along with this, there is frequently a diet that is too low in carbohydrates. The cravings for high-sugar, high-starch foods (cookies and chips and other baked goods) that accompany the compulsive eating are often encouraged by the fact that the client is not eating enough grain-based foods during the day. Low-carb-diet trends today make this easy to do.

Step 5

The body senses that deprivation of carbohydrate and wants to make up for it by the end of the day. I can't tell you how many clients feel they are "good" during the day but over-consume carbs at night. Very often we reverse this trend by adding more healthful grain-based foods during the day. The client's desire for simple carbs (sugar) dies down when the deprivation of these nutritious and delicious foods decreases.

To find out if you might be eating too little carbohydrate, check in with yourself. Does this sound like you?

- You find yourself binge-eating or compulsively eating high-starch or high-sugar foods, particularly in the evening.

- You feel weak and tired, and have less energy for physical activity than you used to.

- You find that it's harder to physically exert yourself two days in a row, as if your muscles take longer to recover than they used to.

- You have cravings for sugar or sweet-grainy foods (like cookies, muffins, bread) that don't just show up as part of a pre-menstrual syndrome.

- You find yourself drooling over your neighbor's plate of pasta or root-vegetable stew and unable to enjoy your own moderately-carb-laden dish. (There's nothing wrong with your lower-carb recipe, by the way. If you were eating enough carbohydrate regularly, then you might not feel so deprived and just enjoy it.)

While other lifestyle or nutritional factors can lead to the above conditions, this is what I find many of my clients complaining about when they are eating too little carbohydrate, particularly foods like rice, potatoes, and other grains. Julia Child was a famous chef who lived near me here in Cambridge, Massachusetts for much of her life and lived to be ninety-two. Anyone who encountered her or watched her top-rated cooking show would not deny that she celebrated the pleasures of food. I started this chapter with her quote, which I'll repeat here because it's so appropriate. "Because of the media hype and woefully inadequate information, too many people nowadays are deathly afraid of their food, and what does fear of food do to the digestive system? I am sure that an unhappy or suspicious stomach, constricted and uneasy with worry, cannot digest properly. And if digestion is poor, the whole body politic suffers." Personally, I think life is too short to spend it being afraid of noodles!

Proteins

Proteins provide the same amount of energy (or calories) as carbohydrates, but this macronutrient provides a more sustained, longer-term energy. Without protein at a meal, we often get hungry an hour or two later, no matter how much food we've eaten. Amino acids, the breakdown components of proteins, are necessary for growth and muscle-building. Most athletes don't want to lose muscle, so they need to get enough protein and carbohydrate in their diets to cover their activity level. We don't need to load up on the protein powders that the bodybuilders will try to sell us, though. Most of us get plenty of protein on a regular basis to maintain or build muscle. Athletes who work out a lot may need more protein and carbohydrate than non-athletes to allow their muscles to recover well between workouts, but it's relatively easy to get that amount of nutrition if an athlete truly listens to hunger cues and just eats more food. Proteins make not only muscles but also organs, hair, nails, hormones, and other vital body substances.

Meats, fish and other seafood, nuts, legumes/dried beans, vegetables, dairy products, and soy-based foods contain protein. Animal sources (meats, fish, and dairy) contain more protein than plant sources (legumes/beans, nuts, vegetables, soy), so we need to eat almost three times as much quantity of plant-based proteins. Vegetarian diets can be very healthy and conscious diets, but some concern about obtaining adequate protein and other minerals that are less available in plants is essential. Discussion of vegetarianism in depth is beyond the scope of this book, though we talk more about this eating lifestyle choice in Step 9.

Fats

Fats are a powerhouse of energy, providing twice as much energy/calories than carbohydrate or protein and providing long-term satiety or fullness. Fats protect our organs, nerves, and neurotransmitter receptor sites in our brains. They assist the absorption of vital fat-soluble vitamins (A, D, E, and K). Fats also give food a pleasurable sensation in our mouths. Women without enough fat in their diets may lose their reproductive function over time. Our brains are made up largely of fat, too. Our brains and neural connections work better when our fat intake is adequate.

Some of my clients and friends and family members have a real craving and full-bodied need for fats, and some seem to be turned off by foods that are extra fatty. I think this is likely temperamental and must be related to what the individual bodies need. Why do some people recoil at the skin and fat on meats while others absolutely love it? Of course, some preferences for certain fats could be environmental and learned. We tend to eat what we are exposed to, and if we've heard negative health messages about eating fattier red meats or chicken skin, we also might avoid these foods. But the true preferences toward or away from certain fats might also be related to differences among bodies. There is interesting new research on the microbiome, outside of the scope of this book, demonstrating that the individual bacterial mix of our guts helps to determine what foods are good for us and which foods are not going to feel as good going down. It's wild to think that gut bacteria could be partly responsible for our food preferences!

Micronutrients

There is much that I could write about all the different types of vitamins and minerals and the foods that contain them. You can find this information easily. In fact, most of the people who come to see me for nutrition therapy know a fair amount about the nutrient content of foods. You probably already know that most fruits contain vitamin C, cruciferous vegetables (kale, collards, and cabbage) have strong anti-cancer properties, and meats and fish contain the most absorbable form of iron. Fruits and vegetables, in particular, are powerhouses of micronutrients (vitamins and minerals) and phytochemicals that have many health-protective qualities. Again, it's beyond the scope of this book to delve into each one. The most important message that I can impart for the journey that we are on together in this book is to eat a wide, colorful variety of foods as much as possible. Doing so ensures that your body receives an abundance of nutrition and health enhancement.

Hopefully, you are working on listening to your body and its unique preferences. Why is it that my body craves certain things at certain times? Why do I love mushrooms so much while other family members shun them? Why do some of my family members seem to choose melons over all other fruits, while I rarely have a taste for cantaloupe? We all have different body chemistries, and I believe that our preferences and leanings give us clues about what nutrition we most need. Of course, environment and deprivation can make us crave things that are emotionally connected and make this confusing. I've seen that when someone's relationship with food improves, those embodied clues truly point to balance, variety, and moderation—and, ultimately, a healthy dose of vitamins and minerals.

Table 1: Nutritional Core Minimum

THE NUTRITIONAL CORE MINIMUM **
CARBOHYDRATES – To Energize

Fruits and Vegetables— 5 units minimum/day	Grains/Starches— 6 units minimum/day
- 1 medium piece of fruit - 1 cup melon - 1/2 cup sliced fruit (grapes, pineapple, etc.) - 1/2 cup fruit or vegetable juice - 1/4 cup dried fruit - 1/2 cup cooked vegetables - 1 cup raw vegetables	- 1/2 cup rice, pasta, quinoa, or other cooked grain - 1 slice sandwich bread or 1/2 sandwich bun - 1/3 large bakery bagel (or 1/2 small store bagel) - 1/2 cup cooked cereal - 1 ounce breakfast cereal (approx. 1/2-1 cup) - 1 small roll, biscuit, or muffin - 5 to 6 small crackers - 2 rice cakes - 1/2 medium potato - 1/2 cup green peas or corn - 3 cups popcorn

PROTEINS – To Sustain

Non-Dairy Proteins—4 units minimum/day	Dairy Proteins—3 units minimum/day (4 units minimum for those age 11-24 and pregnant/breastfeeding women)
- 1 ounce of chicken, turkey, fish, beef, or pork (Note: 3 ounces of meat is about the size of the palm of your hand or a deck of cards) - 2 ounces of shrimp, scallops, crab, lobster - 1/4 cup canned tuna - 1/2 cup cooked beans/legumes - 3 ounces tofu - 1 egg (or 2 egg whites) - 2 rounded tbsp. nut butter - 1/4 cup nuts and/or seeds - 1/2 veggie burger (Note: One unit of protein is approximately equal to 7 grams of protein.)	- 1 cup milk or calcium-fortified soy, almond, rice, or other alternative milk - 1 cup yogurt - 1/2 cup cottage cheese - 1 ounce cheese - 1 ounce ricotta cheese (Note: If you choose not to eat dairy or cannot tolerate it, make sure you add 3-4 more proteins minimum from the non-dairy list, and consider taking a calcium/vitamin D supplement if there are no other rich sources of calcium in your diet.)

** NOTE: THESE ARE ALL MINIMUMS. MOST ACTIVE PERSONS WILL NEED MORE FOOD.

Step 5

FATS—To Satisfy

> Include a source of fat at each meal. Fats are used to round out meals,
> meet energy requirements, and encourage a sense of satiety,
> as well as other important body and brain functions.
>
> Oils (olive, peanut, vegetable, etc.)
> Butter, cream cheese, mayonnaise, hummus
> Occurring naturally in other foods like nuts, avocados,
> olives, cheeses, meats, etc.

Quantity of Food

So how much of these macronutrients and micronutrients do we need to eat, you might ask? Well, that depends on your size, activity level, genetics, metabolism, health status, and many other factors. It's hard to answer this very commonly asked question. In my practice, when someone is clueless about what and how much to eat over the course of a day, I often do a reality check with them around the minimum amount of food we need to eat to receive the nutrients that the body needs on a daily basis. I always advise clients to take even this "core minimum" advice with a grain of salt. However, I review it because I find that many people (especially women) underestimate the amount of food that they need in a given day.

Many of my clients try to eat minimally and end up overeating at other times. It's often eye opening for some to hear that a minimum of six grain units, five fruit and vegetable units, and seven protein units is ideal. And this is just a minimum! Most athletes and even generally active people need more food than this regularly. I also encourage a source of fat at each meal—and ideally some fat at most snacks—to round out meals and provide a sense of fullness that allows us not to think about food for at least a few hours. If hearing information about quantities and portions is uncomfortable for you, please just skip this information. I put it here, again, because I find that it's a helpful reality check for the chronic dieter or restrictive eater who is slowing down their metabolism and depleting their muscle and lean-body tissue by eating too little food.

I want to emphasize that every body's needs and metabolism are different. However, if a client is not getting at least the core minimum nutrients from these main categories, then I can almost guarantee that she does not have enough energy, vitality, and—importantly—resistance to overeating (which is quite a temptation in our culture of food abundance). **When someone asks me what to eat at a meal, I typically and very loosely recommend they have some carb/grain food, some protein food, and some produce (fruit/veg).** We work on that deep body listening to get to know the ratio of each component that works for them, and we use the daily core minimum as a guide. Leaving any of these categories out is likely to create an imbalance over time, but that doesn't mean that we can't eat a meal without protein or grain or fat once in a while and be just fine.

You'll see lots of different "plate" recommendations out there. I don't recommend any particular plate for everyone. I don't believe that all people need to eat the same way, nor do we need to eat the same way each day. If someone needs guidance as to what to put on their plates, in addition to the grain/

protein/produce recommendation, I also recommend that the plate look attractive, tasty, and inviting. I also suggest that the protein take up about one-quarter to one-third of the plate, while the grain/fruits/vegetables take up the other two-thirds to three-quarters. I present here a much more simplistic view of meal planning than you might get from many other sources, but I find this seems to work no matter what your values and preferences are—whether you are eating a more plant-based diet, a vegetarian diet, or are an "opportunivore."

The attractive, tasty, and inviting part can't be underestimated, in my opinion. There is an element of self-care that gets eliminated when we eat food out of its storage containers. However, at times, I also find myself eating in the car or at my desk while checking email. It's inevitable; we can't always eat mindfully with our busy lives, and very often eating while driving or reading is better self-care than not eating. More often than not, though, I recommend trying to give your food the attention it (and we) deserve. I've been known to say to a friend who knows me well, "I need to have a moment with my yummy sandwich. Can I call you back …?"

Other Taste-Oriented Properties of Foods

There are other holistic properties of food beyond nutrition that I don't want to overlook, though nutrition science often ignores them. Eating is a complex experience, and foods have different properties that excite our senses. I'm sure certain foods come to mind when I write the words "Sweet," "Sour," "Bitter," and "Salty." You may or may not have associations with the words "Pungent" or "Astringent." Foods and herbs have these different taste qualities, and many traditions all over the world combine these different flavors to make up the world's cuisines. You may gravitate to certain herbs and flavors based on your constitution. For example, when overheated in the summer sun, many turn to lemonade because lemons are both sour and astringent and feel refreshing. Basil is an herb that is often used in rich, heavy dishes because it supports digestion. If you have an interest in learning about foods, culinary herbs, and how to incorporate this sensory palate into your cooking, I highly recommend Brittany Wood Nickerson's book *Recipes from The Herbalist's Kitchen*, listed at the end of this chapter. My studies of herbalism have increased my appreciation for these sensory properties of food that drive many of our preferences.

Water

Now I must mention the other macronutrient that often gets forgotten: Water. Adequate hydration of our bodies is important. In fact, our bodies are made up of about two-thirds water. Contrary to popular belief, our bodies do a great job of keeping that water balance. In fact, when someone says, "I'm so dehydrated," he probably really means, "I'm so thirsty." Dehydration is life threatening and can land you in a hospital. If we are listening to our thirst, we aren't likely to get dehydrated—even though there is some evidence that thirst signals show up when we are a bit beyond thirsty. Hunger signals register with us sooner than thirst. There has been a lot of debate in the nutrition community about how much hydration is needed. The recommendation for a long time was eight cups of water per day. I always had a hard time believing that a 6'5" basketball player needs the same amount of water as a 5'2" non-athlete. I don't think prescriptions work with fluid any more than prescriptions work with food. Keep in mind that foods have liquid in them (especially fruits and vegetables). Caffeinated beverages used to be called "negative" fluid. Yes, caffeine does make us pee more and lose water, but we can get hydration from a cup of caffeinated tea or coffee. The "negative fluid" theory is not entirely correct.

I will share with you what I tell clients. If you are drinking much less than six to eight cups of fluid (any fluid) per day, try increasing it by a couple of cups. Do you feel any better when you do that—or do you just notice that you pee more and that's it? Also, take a look at your pee. If it's mostly clear (unless you are taking multi-vitamins that give it a bright yellow or greenish tinge), then you are drinking enough. If it's dark yellow, you are likely making your kidneys work harder than you need to and could stand to drink a couple more glasses of water each day. Symptoms of low hydration include tiredness, swollen/stiff joints, headaches, body aches, lightheadedness, poor concentration, constipation, dry mouth/bad breath, and dry skin. These symptoms can be related to other conditions, but it's worth experimenting to see if you feel better after upping your H_2O.

Blood-Sugar Balance

I see people who have chaotic relationships with food making choices that leave them with erratic blood-sugar levels.

If you tend to go long times without something to eat (often followed by eating more than you'd like to at the next meal), then you are probably experiencing a drop in blood sugar that encourages overeating. At the very least, it does not encourage attuned, slow, mindful eating so that you can be aware of your fullness cues.

When you fail to eat when you are hungry, you send your body into a zone of hunger and craving that increases over time. When you ignore hunger—or eat a meal that is not substantial enough to meet your appetite—you stay in that craving zone. You keep thinking about food. Eventually, if you ignore your body's signals more—whether you are doing so on purpose because you are dieting or if you are just rushed and forget to eat—you may get "hangry" and moody. You might feel so hungry that you could bite your best friend's head off, even if she's relatively kind. I call this the "crisis" zone. Your blood sugar is so low that it's hard to get your body to a state of equilibrium. In fact, you could eat an entirely reasonable, balanced meal when you are in "hunger crisis," but it doesn't fill you up or hold you more than an hour or so.

It sounds so basic, but I think this is one of the most frequent eating "mistakes" that I see many of us make around food. I make it myself when I'm in the "focused" zone of a project and don't notice my hunger until it turns ravenous. I've done this a few times while writing this book! Going too long without eating—or eating too-small, less-sustaining meals (like a salad when your body wants a hearty meal) will very often backfire in excessive eating later. The more we make sure that we have enough fuel in our hungry moments—ideally something to eat with carbohydrate, protein, and fat—the more that meal or snack will hold us for a while. Regular eating means we are less likely to think about food more than we want to. We will also sustain energy and blood-sugar levels that will promote balanced eating at the next hunger moment. Hunger is likely to come every three to six hours (depending on the quantity and type of food you eat and your individual metabolism) instead of in hourly bursts and cravings. Eliminating protein and fat in the meal or snack tends to make hunger show up more quickly. Reducing carbohydrate in the meal or snack tends to keep the brain thinking about food—and perhaps craving sugar as a way to take in simple carbs.

I do believe that the single most important nutritional change that most people can make is to eat breakfast within about an hour of waking up and eating sustainable meals and snacks (with carb, protein, and fat) according to hunger throughout the day. Some of my clients need to set a timer regularly during the day to check in with how their hunger is doing so that they don't forget to eat or get too hungry (or "hangry"). Some of my clients agree to eat breakfast as a two-week experiment, knowing they can go back to skipping it after this time. They often never look back because they feel so much less chaotic with food the rest of the day when they start their energy and eating off on the right course. **Regular, attuned eating does not sound like mind-blowing nutritional advice, but it often is. In our distracting, busy world today, this kind of eating sometimes does not feel natural. It will, however, increase your vitality and improve your relationship with food exponentially.**

Meal and Snack Patterns

You don't have to eat three meals per day to eat well. Some people eat four meals per day, and that works better for their energy. They typically eat smaller amounts of food than the three-meal eater or eat two smaller meals. Some people eat only two main meals per day with snacks in between. That works for them. Some people choose to eat mini-meals many times per day, and that satisfies. I caution people against "grazing" too much, because that can keep you constantly thinking about food (when your mind and focus could be engaged in other meaningful pursuits). Also, it can be hard to get all the nutrients that you need if you are relying on portable snacks for most of the day. That said, snacking may be a helpful strategy for eliminating that over-hungry trap when the time between meals is significant. Many Bostonians eat dinner late, so I'm almost always suggesting that clients try a snack around 3:00 or 4:00 p.m. daily. Often that takes the edge off hunger and can prevent binge-eating at night. There might be an emotional trigger for the binge-eating; but if there are also physiological triggers (not enough food all day, too hungry, etc.), then it can be doubly hard to ignore the drive to binge.

For me, having a sense of **abundance** around food has been an important part of my eating-disorder recovery. When I carry food around with me—in my car, in my bag, in my desk drawer—I get the sense that I can eat whenever I need to. I have plenty. And I don't need to eat it all up now because there is going to be enough nearby. In fact, no particular foods are scarce or off-limits for me, aside from an allergy where the consequences of consuming the food far outweigh the benefits. Foods don't have the "charge" that they would if I were to say that I shouldn't have them. This sense of food abundance creates a security that works to keep me healthy and balanced in my enjoyment of food. This stance doesn't necessarily work for everyone, as everyone's underlying issues around food are different. It's an example of a strategy that has worked for me and for others who have had food scarcity—imposed from the outside or by themselves—as part of their eating history. Keeping food closeby and relatively abundant also serves the purpose of keeping me from getting too hungry. And we've already learned how much of a set-up for overeating that can be.

In Step 9, when we get into setting goals and making changes in your eating and other self-care habits, I'll talk more about the decisions many people ask about: Should I eat meat, gluten, dairy? Am I sensitive to certain foods, and how do I figure that out? How do I comb through all the nutrition information that is out there and ultimately listen to my own body when the messages to limit certain foods or food groups are so loud and clear? Can I have a peaceful, healthy relationship with my body and food if I simply eat foods that I like in a balanced way? Isn't that too simple? It is simple. But over and over again, clients who have struggled for decades with every diet find that when they stop dieting, listen to their bodies, and simply eat what they like to eat, moderately, they feel satisfied. Furthermore, their bodies land at the weight they are meant to be. When they stop struggling with their weight and with food in general, then they begin to enjoy eating again. And their bodies feel better because they are tuning in. Ending this struggle is not as easy as it might sound here. There are often emotional obstacles in the way—and the diet or perfect-health mentality is always waiting around every corner to suck you back in.

Nutrition and Health Claims

Author Michael Pollan cites the American Paradox: The more we worry about nutrition, the less healthy we seem to become. I once wrote in my blog that if I see another article about the "Top Ten Foods That You Must Eat to Have Perfect Health," I might just implode. It does drive me crazy to see foods categorized into "good" and "bad," as this perpetuates the myth that there is one more noble way to eat than another. Pollan proposes a new (and ancient) answer to the question of what we should eat that comes down to seven simple but liberating words: *Eat food. Not too much. Mostly plants.* By urging us to eat food, he challenges the prevailing nutrient-by-nutrient approach—what he calls "nutritionism"—and proposes an alternative way of eating informed by the traditions and ecology of real, well-grown, unprocessed food. Our health, he argues, cannot be divorced from the health of the food chains of which we are a part.

Yes, I am a registered dietitian, and I know that some foods have more vitamins, minerals, and beneficial phytochemicals than others. I know that the more colorful plate of food is the most nutrient dense. I'm not going to argue that encouraging us to get more fruits and veggies in our diets is wrong. However, encouraging people to believe that drinking a green smoothie each day makes up for erratic and unbalanced eating the rest of the week is a grave mistake. I have seen too many intelligent people skip meals and crash because they believed that drinking a smoothie was a substitute for listening to their body's needs and preferences and hunger.

So, I hate to burst any bubbles, but here is the real deal about smoothies and quinoa and kale (and whatever the health food of the week might be). They aren't perfect foods. In fact, *no one food* is perfect. Please give up that view. Our bodies need lots of different nutrients and foods to be healthy. Full disclosure: I actually like quinoa—and kale—and frequently make smoothies of many types. My favorite has berries, banana, nut butter, freshly grated ginger, chocolate (cacao), and almond milk in it. My children will sometimes catch me sneaking some spinach into their fruit smoothies, and they don't generally mind because there are also plenty of sweet-tasting berries in there, too. Fruits, vegetables, legumes, coconut, whole grains, avocados ... Yes, these are all health-giving foods that may have disease-preventative qualities. What I worry about is the way that we give health-improving foods such rock-star status, and they start showing up all over the place.

For instance, we used to think that coconut oil was on the "bad" list and clogged our arteries. Then, a more recent bit of research indicated that coconut might be quite good for us. Now it's showing up in everything from yogurt to flours to bottled coconut water drinks. None of those processed foods are bad for us by themselves, but we don't know what the effect of eating umpteen coconut derivatives in one day might be. Many of these products are not coconut-the-way-nature-intended. I once did a diet assessment of a vegetarian client years ago and found out that she was eating seven different products with derivatives of soy in them in one day. (This is pretty easy to do with all of the soybean oil and added soy protein in many foods.) Everything that she'd read was telling her that soy was super healthy for her, but I still cautioned her against so much processed soy. Highly fortified foods are still highly processed foods. And, though I believe that we can enjoy all foods in moderation, I'm fairly sure that anxiously trying to eat the most nutrient-dense diet is not so good for our digestion. It's the "anxiously" part that has increased in the last couple of decades. We either forget that food is a pleasure or we feel the conflict when we see the covers of the women's magazines that have large photos of yummy treats right next to headlines about how to start your new year's diet. Again, the message is "Food is Love, but don't eat too much." *Mangia, mangia*—but don't get too plump.

We take nutritional advice to the extreme not only because moderation isn't that fun. We sometimes aim to eat virtuously to feel better about ourselves—and feel in control of our lives in an increasingly complex world. **Whenever we listen to the "Top Ten Foods You Can't Do Without" and stop listening to our inner wisdom about what our bodies most need to eat at any given moment, we create a big disconnect between our bodies and the act of eating. We trust someone else's advice for how we should eat instead of our own—and we** believe, erroneously, that there is a food prescription out there that everyone should follow. Studies have shown that young children, over the course of a week and month (though not daily), will naturally choose a diet that is varied and complete nutritionally. When I once asked my then-eight-year-old daughter why she didn't eat a particular meal, she said, "Because I didn't like it," looking at me like I must be crazy if I think that she's going to eat anything that she doesn't like. She would also sometimes say, "I don't like this, but I'm really hungry, so I'm eating it." A young child's logic is pretty simple around food when it hasn't been tainted by the "shoulds" and "should-nots" out there.

The antidote to all the conflicting health and nutrition messages is mindful eating with nutritional common sense. This kind of eating is not as simple or easy as it sounds for some, but it's how many of us used to eat as children until the adults around us gave us reasons to think outside our bodies about what to eat. Relearning to eat in a mindful, embodied way can be profoundly liberating and nourishing. Combine it with mindful, conscious movement (Step 6), and you are on your way to having a connected, well-nourished, and well-cared-for body and self.

References and Resources:

Tribole, E. and Resch, E. *Intuitive Eating: A Revolutionary Program That Works.* New York, NY: St. Martin's Press, 2012.

Nickerson, B.W. *Recipes from the Herbalist's Kitchen: Delicious, Nourishing Food for Lifelong Health and Well-Being.* North Adams, MA: Storey Publishing, 2017.

Pollan, M. *In Defense of Food: An Eater's Manifesto.* New York, NY: Penguin Books, 2008.

STEP 6
Conscious, Joyful Movement

A pause is, by nature, time limited. We resume our
activities, but we do so with increased presence and
more ability to make choices. In the pause before sinking
our teeth into a chocolate bar, for instance, we might
recognize the excited tingle of anticipation, and perhaps
a background cloud of guilt and self-judgment. We may
then choose to eat the chocolate, fully savoring the taste
sensations, or we might decide to skip the chocolate and
instead go out for a [walk]. When we pause, we don't
know what will happen next. But by disrupting our
habitual behaviors, we open to the possibility of new and
creative ways of responding to our wants and fears.

~ Tara Brach, *Radical Acceptance*

I open Step 6 with this quote from Tara Brach because I
think it encapsulates some of the other steps we've already

visited on this journey. It also introduces the topic of **mindful, conscious, joyful movement**. Conscious, joyful movement is not just some woo-woo, psycho-babble terminology for exercise. I make a clear distinction between the type of exercise regimen that the Fitbits of the world prescribe and the kind of activity that we engage in because our bodies and minds desire and ask to move. In fact, if you are walking just to get a thumbs-up from your handheld device, then that is probably going to get old fast. I think that's why so many of my daughters' middle school peers are wearing their parents' dusty step-counters. It's a bit like the skyrocketing gym enrollment on January 1st, followed by dwindling attendance by March 1st.

I'm not entirely poo-poo-ing step-counters or the stairs-to-nowhere (well, maybe I am), but I do think they encourage people to move for the wrong reasons. If your efforts to be physically active are all about looking good, weighing less, getting a thumbs-up, or competing for the most steps with your co-workers, then, once the initial thrill of doing something new wears off, why bother? Physical activity is truly about being in your body (ideally, getting a break from being in your mind) and being in the present. If the workout feels good and is fun and engaging, you'll be more likely do it again and again. Maybe for decades. If the exercise is tedious, exhausting, punishing, or completely attached to an external prescription (steps walked, calories burned, etc.), then it's not aligned with what your body wants at that very moment. The movement might be boring or (worse) compulsive. In my experience, people who maintain regular physical activity throughout their lives do so because they like to move. They've found ways to move their bodies that feel good and drop them joyfully into the present moment. I call this "mindful movement."

I regularly dance because my body and spirit miss it when I don't dance, and they let me know about it. I feel restless, disconnected from my self, and a real desire to leap from deep within myself. I find joy in moving my body to music. My communicative, busy mind loves the challenge of dancing in nonverbal partnership with others. But when I'm tired after a too-long day of work, or I'm fighting off the latest cold virus circulating through my family, I stay put. I listen to my body's wisdom, even if it's different this week. No Fitbit or rigid exercise schedule allows for that break; only *you* can give yourself that important rest when you pay attention to what your body needs.

My ninety-four-year-old grandmother never touched a gym, but she kept going all these years because she valued a clean house and got into the "zone" (the present moment) by sweeping and dusting. I mentioned earlier that her husband, my grandfather, walked the golf course himself into his early nineties while the "young guys" rode the golf carts. He didn't do this because he was trying to keep himself svelte. He did this because not using a golf cart made him feel strong, capable, and his version of a badass on the golf course. Take care of your body like we hope to take care of this planet: With an eye on sustainability.

Many of my clients exercise compulsively. They can't take a day off without tremendous guilt and self-flagellation. When I dig deeper, they often don't even really like the exercise that they are doing. Running hurts their knees, or yoga makes them feel incompetent around all the young pretzel-types. Somewhere they got into their heads how much exercise they needed to do in a week. They stick to it religiously. That's fine if it lines up with what feels good in their bodies and their life falls nicely into place around that schedule; but so often I hear about hours of sleep lost, social engagements declined, and injuries worsened because the workout program was literally in charge. The joy of moving the body gets stripped from the activity when it becomes compulsive.

Does this sound like you?

I feel wrong if I don't run six miles, but after I do that, I am completely wiped out and exhausted the rest of the day,

or

I should be exercising more, but I feel demoralized going into the gym, so I do nothing, or I walked three miles today, but that doesn't feel like enough.

In each of these cases, my clients want to move, but they are moving according to some prescription that they hold in their heads—or that a well-meaning health professional or parent or friend handed to them. What they aren't doing is listening to their own bodies' wisdom about how much activity is enough or right for them.

Let's take the example of the runner who feels compelled to run so many miles per day but whose body is not recovering well from it. Marathon runners know that training requires lots of running, as well as lots of calories from food. If you are running your planned number of miles but feeling exhausted instead of energized, then you are probably running more than your self-care and feeding will allow. Are you eating enough food and sleeping enough hours to sustain and support that level of running, particularly if it's daily? You may be surprised by just how many calories and sleep runners need to repair all the muscle fibers and tissues that break down and build up with regular running. In fact, if we don't eat enough calories, we can't build muscle doing any physical activity. Muscle-building is anabolic, which means that it requires extra food above and beyond the food that our bodies need to survive and function well.

If your body is getting enough food and enough sleep, and you are not training beyond your body's capacities, then you should be able to recover from your physical activity and feel good (albeit a little sore) the next day. If your exercise routine is wiping you out, then it's time to take a look at your eating and other habits. Maybe your busy lifestyle is tiring enough, and exercising every other day would be more sustainable than daily workouts. Maybe two times per week is sufficient for you right now. Just because the Surgeon General makes particular recommendations doesn't mean that the advice is suitable for every person under every circumstance. Take a look at what level of exertion and frequency your lifestyle can handle. Try eating more if you feel like you aren't recovering well between workouts. Many of my clients are surprised that just adding more food (often carbohydrates) gives them more energy and helps their bodies recover better from physical activity.

High-intensity exercise like running is certainly not for every body. Nor is going to a gym. The person I quoted above who felt humiliation and shame going to a gym was not choosing the right form of movement for her. Often when I interview someone about their exercise habits, I ask them to name ways of moving their body that feel good. If going to the gym feels satisfying, so be it. For many, however, gym exercises become boring, repetitive, and something to dread. Finding forms of movement that motivate and feel fun will sustain interest. Walking outside will often feed the senses (and fulfill our hunger for nature) much more than staring at a TV in a gym. Clients of mine have discovered yoga, kayaking, swimming, dancing, martial arts, gardening, and other forms of movement that help them feel more connected to their bodies and the joy of movement. One of my clients joined a women's hockey league and found it exhilarating and fun. The treadmill just wasn't doing it for her anymore.

I once had an injury and needed to do some physical therapy and strengthening as my knee and hip healed. I hate traditional strength training, even though I know that it's good for my body. I find it boring, and it feels pointless to me at the moment, so I have no interest in sustaining it, even though I want to have a healthy, able body as I continue to age. Put me in a kayak or on my bicycle, but don't make me lift a dumbbell or ride a bike that's nailed to the ground! During my injury recovery, Peter Benjamin, the practitioner who helped me out, made strength work fun. He taught me exercises that I could do with my daughters around the house. He threw heavy balls back and forth with me. (Playing ball is way more fun than lifting weights!) Peter made the experience of strengthening and healing fun and interactive. I'm so grateful for that experience and for what it taught me about what I need to keep movement a joyful part of my life.

I often hear clients say that they did some walking, or they worked an eight-hour shift on their feet, or they did some stretching and yoga—but *"it's not enough."* Enough for whom, I ask? Sometimes we have unrealistic expectations about how much movement is "enough." Our bodies benefit when we ride our bikes to the store, walk from the subway station to work, wait on tables or patients, and dance around the yard with a toddler. You might get up from your desk if you sit a lot (set an alert on your computer if you need to) and stretch and move in the way that makes your body feel good. If you tune in, your body will likely tell you what it wants. Find ways to be creative and move spontaneously in your life, so that scheduling exercise doesn't have to be a chore or another to-do list item.

And let it be enough.

Emily is learning how to move mindfully. She tells me that she ran a few errands outside on this gorgeous day in the late afternoon. Emily walked for about twenty minutes total. Since she sits at her computer most of the day, she attended to her body by unrolling the yoga mat that she keeps in her office and stretching out her back and hamstrings. She also did some physical-therapy exercises that she was recently given to prevent a recurring injury. It was not a long exercise session. This movement was not significant aerobic, strength, or flexibility work, but it was just right for Emily on a day when she had already worked a fair amount. She told me that she felt good in her body afterward—energized, rejuvenated, and not wiped out. She had enjoyed the autumn leaves and the fluffy clouds on her errands and out her window while she stretched. After a short meditative rest (Shavasana) to close her movement activities, she went back to her desk chair. After this bit of action and mind-clearing, she was able to sit down, feel creative, and write a draft of the blog post that she wanted to write before the end of her workday. Emily is learning to move in the way that works for her particular day and her lifestyle. She may do some more vigorous exercise on her weekends, but this workday routine was nourishing and so different from her all-or-nothing belief that she had to pound the pavement or get no exercise at all.

Our bodies mean to move, yet we sit and stare at screens more and more these days. We need to be active more than ever; but if we mindlessly exercise (not listening to our bodies and what they are telling us about what feels right and what feels lousy), then we can develop a challenging relationship with physical activity. About a year ago, I told the next story on my blog. I think it bears repeating here because it demonstrates my own journey with conscious, joyful movement.

Two years ago, I took my first ballet class in almost two decades. Believe it or not, it was heavenly. It felt like a home-coming. And, of course, my forty-five-year-old body was very different than the body of my youth. I was surprised, though, by how much my body remembered ballet. The sequences. The patterns. The steps. The turnout. In fact, it was a wise clinician treating me for a recurring hip/knee injury who noticed that my kneecaps are not in the same place as most people's knees. The dance training that took up most of my free time from age six to twenty-six encouraged my bones and joints to develop differently: Quite turned out, compared to most people's joints. Although the yoga of today was keeping me strong in some ways, it was torquing my limbs, forcing my joints and bones into parallel positions that were just not normal for them.

When I started turning my feet gently out in yoga class, the instructors corrected me. Sometimes they corrected me many times. Once I explained to the teachers that to put my knees over my toes, which is proper alignment for a yoga pose, I had to turn my feet out a bit and showed them my kneecaps; they got it. At least some of them did. I look rather weird in a yoga class, but thank goodness I don't care much. And I find it a challenge to work with my strange anatomy. An osteopath also told me that the natural way for our skeletons to stand up is with a slightly open turnout, not parallel. (So much for mountain pose.) And my own particular grounding stance is even more turned out at the hips than average because of my young dance training. These two healing women providers were edging me back to ballet dancing as a way that is natural for my particular body to move. I know I'll never go back to *pointe* shoes. (Heck, I barely ever wear heels. I vowed never to torture my feet again.) But here I was being pointed back to ballet for several different reasons, and I was unsure about how it would be to try a class after twenty years.

I wondered if I actually could dance with "Beginner's Mind." Also, could I go to class with my body as it is right now: Older, less flexible, post-childbirth? Surprisingly, I did. The piano started playing. With my first *plié*, I felt that old, familiar grace. My arms and legs did what they had done thousands of times before. Many years had passed between my younger dancing days and today; I felt different. I was stronger in some places in my body and weaker in others. My brain and body did not coordinate as fast as they did when I was a young dancer. But I felt the same exhilarated stirring inside of me. Something almost spiritual. I felt strangely at home.

As the class progressed, it got more challenging, and I had to exert more effort. I became more aware of just how out of shape I was (at least for a ballerina). Some combinations were beyond my coordination. I laughed at myself when my feet got twisted up. And I cheered myself on if I finally got the formation right. And that's when it dawned on me that I was indeed returning to ballet with Beginner's Mind—and Heart. I was kinder to myself. When I knew that I didn't look like the seasoned, regular dancers in the class, I just reminded myself that, for a forty-five-year-old with two kids who hasn't taken a class in twenty years, I was doing just amazing. I found myself talking to myself inside, like I would to one of my daughters or a client: "Good for you for trying." "This will get easier with more practice." "Look at what you *can* do!"

I remember talking to myself when I was a young dancer, particularly when I was in my teens. I was hard on myself. I pushed myself to have flatter splits, higher kicks, bigger leaps. I compared myself endlessly to the other, presumably better, dancers. I said punishing things to myself when I messed up the dance steps; I did not laugh with amusement like I was doing today. I did not accept that overextending my legs is not so kind. I once was very hard on myself and hard on my body. It's no surprise that this self-critical teen developed an eating disorder. I struggled with bulimia, binge-eating, and restricting food until I finally got sick of it all and worked on my recovery.

I was one of the lucky ones who got sick young and got well relatively fast, with the help of good people and a strong desire to move forward in my life. I danced ballet, and eventually modern dance, through my recovery and college and did find a kinder way to view my more grown-up body and self.

I had been recovered for many years when I decided to stop ballet at age twenty-six. I was taking adult classes with the Boston Ballet while working in the city and then switched to a smaller adult class in my hometown outside the city. My study of dance took a back seat to my work and other facets of my life. Somehow, though, I found that if I didn't dance, I missed connecting with a large part of my soul. So, I started to find other forms of dance that were fun and joyful for me: Swing, barefoot boogie, African, and contact improvisation. Other, freer dance forms were calling to me and encouraging my self-expression in ways ballet never had. Swing dance is a very improvisational dance style, and I had a lot of fun with that. African dance spoke to my spiritual connection with nature. Contact improvisation, a partner dance form that involves shared weight, really cracked me open. The contact-improv community is quite different from the ballet community, and the dance form felt really *alive* to me. It called me to be in the moment. No choreography. Just whatever arises between a dancer and the floor and the partners that come along. Instead of following a prescribed sequence of steps that someone else taught me and I memorized, I was creatively moving in real time. It was so much fun to see what arose!

Starting in my late twenties, I felt the pull away from structured, rigid dance forms and found my own creative expression.

At the same time, I got more creative in my work with clients. I looked more critically at many things in my life. In many ways, I started to dance to the beat of my own drum. Eventually, it was contact improvisation and a curiosity about dancing on stilts that introduced me to David, my current partner and truest love. So, it was with consciousness that I decided to give up ballet and never look back. Until now.

Why now? As I explained earlier, two clinical opinions told me that my hips and knees move better in turnout than parallel and that certain parts of my body needed strengthening. While I had to reject choreographed dance to find my own creative voice in movement—and probably in my life in my twenties and thirties—I could now, in my mid-forties, return to choreography and rhythm and routine with new respect and a stronger sense of self. Today I know well and honor my body's limitations and preferences.

I haven't rejected the more improvisational dance forms with my return to ballet. I enjoy being spontaneous and creative in my body more than anything. DJ-ing a dear friend's fiftieth birthday was one of my music and dance highlights of the last several years. Creative expression and dance are important to me, and they allow me to write and practice nutrition therapy with fluidity and fresh energy every day. But I don't need to fully reject ballet anymore, a dance form that trained my body to move in certain ways and still feels grounding and familiar. In fact, it connects me to a younger part of myself. Instead of focusing on the aesthetic of ballet, I find myself just being present in the sheer joy of moving.

I am also in a very different place around Step 2: Body Acceptance. I am not used to dancing with mirrors anymore, and I found myself forgetting that there were mirrors on one of the walls of the studio. Every once in a while, I would glance at myself in the mirror and be surprised at what I saw. I look at myself now in a very matter-of-fact way, with far less judgment than I did as a young dancer. I feel how different my relationship with the mirror is today. I feel reverence for my older, able body. I feel respect and not criticism.

My comparing mind doesn't shut off completely; instead, I notice several people who are also on the wrong foot, like I am. I choose to focus my attention very differently and less critically. I decide to move across the floor with some of the talented dancers because I know I can "follow the leader" behind them. When I was a younger ballet dancer, I wouldn't dare do that because I didn't want to look clumsy next to more graceful, capable dancers. As an older woman, I dance across the floor with others with much less ego than I used to have. I am always surprised at how different and liberating this feels.

I also don't push my body too much. Sometimes I feel a little sore the next day, as if I have used muscles that I don't use regularly. But I don't feel some of the more stabbing pains that I sometimes felt in my joints after I did yoga. Pain- and injury-free two years later, I truly believe the clinicians who told me that perhaps ballet suits my body better than yoga does. Returning to even one dance class per week has helped to heal all of my alignment challenges, particularly if I am listening to my body as I practice. How interesting it was for me to learn that a form of dance that not only was a childhood joy for me but, in some ways, also encouraged my teenage eating disorder, could now heal my body thirty years later!

The experience of dancing ballet again also showed me how far I have come in improving my relationship with my body and self. How amazing it feels to connect with that younger part of me and treat her more kindly and gently. How freeing it was to return to ballet class for the sheer joy of moving with flowing grace to live piano. I focused on the pleasure, feeling my body grow stronger and more fluid. How grounding it was to feel at home in my body, despite its limitations and battle scars and history, and to just appreciate the things that it can do. How healing it is to respect and feel grateful for a body that can move in some of the ways that it always moved as a child—a child who loved, more than anything, to dance.

- **What form of movement nourishes and feels good to your body and soul?**

- **Do you like to move outside or inside—or a combination of both, depending on the weather?**

- **Do you like to move your body alone or with others?**

- **Do you have more energy for physical activity in the morning, afternoon, or evening?**

- **How does movement fit best into the rest of your life?**

- **Does vigorous or more gentle action really ground you? Or a combination of both—perhaps depending on the day?**

Step 6

My advice for cultivating mindful, conscious, joyful movement:

- **Find ways to move that you love and that help you feel present and accepting of your amazing, unique body.**

- **Listen to your body. If you feel too sore, tired, and spent after exercising, you may be doing too much at a level that is not sustainable—or your daily-activities plate may be too full for that level of physical activity.**

- **Never ignore injuries. Soreness, when you use new muscles, is normal, but pain is a message from your body. What is it trying to tell you?**

- **Think outside the box (or gym). Find ways to move in your daily life. And, yes, taking the stairs and walking or biking downtown does count! What little forms of mindful, joyful movement can you add into your busy life to provide nourishing-movement nuggets?**

And if your body doesn't feel so good moving at first—if it's been a while or your body has changed and you don't feel as able as you once did—then it's even more important that you find something that you enjoy on some level. You may need to move regularly for a while to get to a place of ease and comfort—let alone joy. Sometimes clients with a trauma history or who live in higher-weight bodies avoid movement and exercise because it protects them from feeling shame. Sometimes personal trainers or individual movement/yoga therapists who are versed in trauma work and/or Health-At-Every-Size can be encouraging support on this journey. Make sure that if you are moving with others or with a trainer, you don't lose that connection with your own body. (Hopefully, good instructors/movement therapists will assist with this.) Our bodies tell us when we've had enough or when we need to do something different. Stretching with a trainer can be good for the body; but mindful stretching, in which you follow the needs that your body is indicating, may be even more nourishing. Refresh yourself with Step 4, and do some of that Deep Listening to your body while you move and stretch and play. Slow down, and notice what your body likes. It may surprise you!

I don't know about you, but the right music can transform dish washing into a satisfying dance party in my kitchen. Movement comes in all shapes and sizes. If you find a way to move that you love, you will be more likely to continue. Movement is like eating: It is a pleasure that sustains us and should remind us that being in a body is one of the joys of life. Honor your body's wisdom. What kind of movement are you hungry for—today, in this moment?

Oh, and one last point. Please, remember that your body is just one facet of your Self. A spirit, a soul is within you, and that is your truest nature. Your body (or the way you choose to adorn your body) may reflect your values and spirit, but your body is not who you are. When my clients become more whole-self-focused and less body-focused, they eat in a way that aligns with their own self-care, and they move in ways that feel right and feed their souls. In the next Step, we'll dive into connecting with that core self and its values to create sustaining self-care practices and set goals.

STEP 7

Clarify Values to
Live a Life You Love

Don't worry about what the world needs. Ask what
makes you come alive, and do that, because what
the world needs is people who have come alive.

~Howard Thurman

We have explored eating and moving quite a bit up
to this point. Hopefully, you are feeling a little more
spaciousness because you are less worried about food and your
body and feeling more ease. Maybe you aren't quite there yet.
That's okay. It's a process—for some, a lifelong process. These
Steps are not linear and will typically be revisited. Step 7 is a
gear shift and focuses on clarifying values.

What does this have to do with healing my relationship
with food, you might ask? Well, not only can defining values
help you with food, exercise, and self-care decisions, but values

clarification can make so many things in life clearer. When you know yourself and what is important to you, then you get clearer on decisions and choices multiple times per day. This means that you find clarity about what is important to you as a unique individual. This may be different than what is important to your peer group or community or parents or spouse. You don't disconnect from those communities and loved ones—you simply have a lens that you can look through to make your most aligned choices. It's a lens that shows you what gives you vitality and energy. If you look inside yourself and figure that out, then you don't need that coffee or green smoothie or dark chocolate to give it to you. Those may be good choices on a day when you didn't get quite enough sleep, but connecting the moments of your day to your core values provides a different kind of energy, one that energizes on a level that no one food or supplement or yoga pose can.

Figuring out what's important to you is not as easy as it sounds. Many of my clients come to see me for the first time without a sense of what they need most in life. I didn't have a real sense of this myself until I was in my thirties, and I keep revisiting my core values and needs every year or so. I notice how much they change as I grow and experience life differently over time.

There are many values-clarification exercises and multiple lists of core values and needs out there. I'm choosing a list here from Russ Harris's **Acceptance and Commitment Therapy (ACT)** work that I find is a good place to start. (See Table 1.) If you'd like more exhaustive lists of core values and needs, you can find them by doing a simple search. I have found, however, that it's useful to have a smaller list to start and to notice the things that might be missing for you. Chances are, those items are essential to you. For instance, one values list I came across had "beauty/aesthetics" on it but not "nature." I discovered that this must be a core value of mine that requires tending to. I find beauty, repose, and inner strength in nature—either through a walk in the woods among the incredible tapestry of tree growth, or the simple abundance of a flower, or a bunch of herbs from my garden that I gather inside to make tea. I know that if I go too long without regular exposure to the beauty of nature, I feel kind of dead inside. It's consistently been a core value for me that I need to "feed" regularly.

What feeds you? Remember, there are hundreds of different values, and I have listed only the most common ones. An exercise that you might find both challenging and fun is choosing your top ten values and then narrowing that down further to your top three. Not all of the values on the list will be relevant to you, and sometimes it helps to cross out the ones that don't resonate first. Keep in mind that there are no "right" or "wrong" values. If I like little yellow cherry tomatoes best and you like the big red ones, that doesn't mean that my taste in vegetables is better than yours. We're just different in our tastes. We might also have different values. And, personally, I believe these differences between people keep life interesting. Take some time to explore the list in Table 1, and notice which values resonate more for you. I strongly recommend that you take some time to do this exercise. Connecting with our deepest longings helps us to make choices aligned with them (Step 9), and this ultimately enhances our lives.

When my clients make more choices from this deep, core place, something amazing happens. They don't use food as much—either compulsively overeating or obsessively under-eating. As I said in the Introduction of this book, food is one of our most basic human needs. It's one of the first needs that we communicated as an infant. No wonder food gets into the mix when we are not attending to our core needs and desires. **I see this over and over again: Simultaneously, clients get in touch with their values and needs and begin to start asking for what they need from themselves, from others, and from life. When this happens, food gradually comes into balance. I more easily feed my body what it needs when I'm also attending to the greater needs in my life.**

In the Boston area, I facilitate therapeutic book clubs called "The No Diet Book Clubs," which are little recovery communities. Members read books on mindful, intuitive eating and living together and support each other in their journeys to heal their relationships with food, body, and self. One day, one of my groups discussed the ways that we can be afraid sometimes to sit still and ask ourselves what fills us up. We struggle to ask, "What nourishes my heart and soul?" We compulsively eat, drink, shop, exercise, text, clean, play games. We are—all of us, and I am far from perfect here—sometimes afraid to just sit still, simply be, and check in with our hearts. I wonder if we are sometimes afraid of what we might find. We fear that we don't know what our heart's desire is. Or if we do know what it is, we don't know the first thing about connecting to it or bringing it into our lives. My group agreed that it's much easier just to keep (insert food behavior, be it binge-eating, restricting, or eating carelessly) than to change and do something else—even if that something else might be good for us. Some of us are so conditioned to feel lousy, criticize ourselves, and live in our heads instead of our hearts, that it is hard to imagine operating otherwise. Change is hard. We need support and strength to do things differently.

I know that clients are moving toward a full recovery from disordered eating (no matter their path to get there) when they begin to truly cultivate the things that help them to feel connected to themselves—and their unique values and purpose. Do you experience that groundedness and that sense that all is well in the world when you feel the passion behind a particular activity? Doesn't your life just flow better when you are feeding your spirit and senses—and when you find moments of truly being in the present? It might be spending time in nature or with a trusted friend or meditating or getting lost in a project that excites you.

In those moments, you are not thinking endlessly about things that already happened or worrying about things in the future that are beyond your control. You are living in the present moment. Doesn't life just flow better for you when you connect with an activity that resonates with you? Do you feel a little relief from the thinking, analyzing part of your brain? You are likely not worrying about what you just ate or what you are going to eat later—or your future health as a result of any of your choices. You are probably not thinking about food at all, at least until your body gives you the clear signal that it's time to refuel. Some of us find these moments of just being present more easily than others. Be patient with your own, personal journey.

In addition to completing a values assessment—either the one in this book or another—I invite you to ask yourself this important question:

> *What fills* ME *up? What nourishes my soul and spirit and keeps me grounded in the present?*

Some answers from clients recently include: listening to music, praying or meditating, walking in nature, taking care of someone they love or their home, dancing, hanging out with friends, or playing with a pet. In fact, animals are especially helpful at keeping us in the present. They don't know any better. It's what they do and where they live.

Explore and discover what makes you feel happy, present, and full right now. You may find that eating becomes less of a battle and big deal when you feed your soul adequately. **And sometimes the binge-eating or food obsessing or exercise resistance will creep back in here and there. I recommend trying to notice compassionately all the self-criticism that comes back with it. See these setbacks as a sign that your soul and spirit need more nourishment.** Don't be afraid to sit quietly and ask your heart what it needs if you find yourself hanging out with food that you don't want to eat—or agonizing about what to choose on a menu because you are afraid to eat what you really want. Be gentle with yourself, and explore what you are hungering for. Perhaps it's one of those core values that is calling for more attention.

Another note about emotional needs, in particular. When we can't seem to get our needs met, then we sometimes look for substitutes. We create strategies to feel better about ourselves or win approval. They can include compulsive achievement or the serving of others to win the attention that we desire. They can include obsessively trying to achieve a certain look or weight. Other strategies to get our needs met might include the more instant gratification that food, alcohol, or drugs provide. Of course, the pleasure is temporary, but these strategies work—at least in the moment. Unfortunately, many strategies that provide pleasure, relief, or attention don't work in the long run and may create more suffering. Many of my clients try to compensate for compulsive overeating by restricting food. Then, the cycle starts again, as the food deprivation creates the wanting that fuels the strategy (overeating). As we become more consistent with using food behaviors as a strategy, we move farther away from understanding—and more effectively meeting—our deepest needs.

We all need love and belonging. We also have lots of other kinds of needs. See Table 2 for a list of universal human needs. I find it helpful to notice that we *all* have these basic needs. Take a look at the list, and examine which needs are most critical for you—at this moment, in this week, in your life in general. Notice that there is some overlap in the values list in Table 1 and the needs list in Table 2. Marshall Rosenberg, author of the best-selling book and widely practiced art of *Nonviolent Communication,* asserts that underlying needs are behind all human beings' actions. Sometimes it's not so obvious what the need is, but I highly recommend exploring this concept more, if you are interested. Being able to identify the needs behind any action can build compassion for both yourself and for others.

Here's an example that involves a choice around food and may make applying Step 7 in such choices clearer. Roberta described a dilemma she felt while eating in an airport. She prefers to eat free-range, organic chicken for environmental and health reasons. The only option in the airport that looked remotely appealing and nourishing enough for how hungry Roberta felt was a wrap sandwich that contained chicken. She knew it was highly unlikely that this restaurant carried organic, free-range chicken, and she wanted to know what she "should" have done. I told her that only she could answer that question. We defined Roberta's conflict and erased the "should" from the equation. (This is one of my favorite exercises. I hate "shoulds.") The conflict had occurred in her mind. On one side, she valued eating a certain way and preferred to choose sources of humanely raised meat. Her desire to take care of her body and what she put into it was behind this practice, as well as her concern for the animals and our planet. On the other side, she had learned, after many years of failed diets, that she benefits on many levels when she eats in a balanced, health-sustaining way. For her, this means balanced meals with substantial protein in them, choosing foods that she likes. She desires to care for her body and soul by doing so.

Roberta was in a dilemma, a conflict. She had two opposing needs, and she also needed to eat. She could have chosen the sandwich or something else. That, ultimately, doesn't matter. Really. What is important is that she was able to notice the conflict and resolve it somehow. She didn't give her food choice too much power to make her feel virtuous or bad, wrong or right. She made a decision and was able to live with it. The fact that she needed to check in with me about whether it was "OK" or not, though, speaks to the work that she still has to do in learning to trust herself. Roberta does know how to feed herself well, but she wanted to make sure that she hadn't made a wrong choice. Again, there are no bad or good decisions. Only choices, made either consciously or unconsciously. There was no question that Roberta had made a conscious food choice, taking her values, needs, and desires into account. What food she chose didn't ultimately matter. She would either feel good in her body and mind and move on, or not feel so good and learn from it for the next time these competing needs came up again. No judgment—just noticing and learning from the dilemma.

We operate best—in our food decisions as well as in bigger life decisions—when we operate from a frame of reference that is inside ourselves, honoring *our* truths and hungers and preferences instead of those of the people around us. If an office worker recognizes that her body wants warm, grounding food and chooses the hearty soup, she will feel centered and soothed all afternoon. If she had grabbed the salad, like everyone else around her who was dieting, she might be left feeling hungry, distracted, and unsatisfied afterwards. If an athlete is listening to his values about sustainability in his sport, he is more likely to notice that twinge in his knee and stop, instead of pushing on through pain and hurting himself. If we all listen to our hearts and our bodies, as well as aim to create a life that holds meaning and enjoyment for us, then we can say "No" to the things that don't resonate with the life that we want. We can also say "Yes" to the things and people that line up with our values and dreams.

Geneen Roth said in her book *Women, Food, and God*, "If you wait to respect yourself until you are at the weight you imagine you need to be to respect yourself, you will never respect yourself, because the message you will be giving yourself as you reach your goal is that you are damaged and cannot trust your impulses, your longings, your dreams, your essence at any weight."[1] As we clarify our values and get in touch with what's important to us in our lives, the importance of being a certain weight or eating a certain number of calories or eating clean doesn't matter that much. It all seems so insignificant when our values are justice or service or family or love.

Samantha, who is recovering from anorexia nervosa, told me that she wished she'd understood that she might be using food to keep from figuring out what her values and needs are. She started to realize that focusing on food and her body was "safer" and more familiar. "I used my eating disorder to distract me from life because I was scared of it." For example, Samantha now realizes that one of her core values is creativity. There is more at stake if she fails at one of her creative projects than if she simply doesn't drink the right smoothie. She says, "I wish I'd had this awareness happen sooner—this awareness of the distraction of food and what it was doing to my life and keeping me from. For others, I hope it will come before ten-plus years of not understanding what the whole cycle is about."

Sometimes it's safer to stay in the eating-disorder mindset, the obsession with food, the addictive process, instead of facing

---

[1] Reprinted with permission of Scribner, a division of Simon and Shuster, Inc. from *Women, Food, and God* by Geneen Roth. Copyright 2010 by Geneen Roth Associates, Inc. All rights reserved.

the unmet needs underneath. Sometimes there is a lot of pain and loss that comes from recognizing those unmet needs. If you discover this yourself, give yourself some time with this process. Don't be afraid to receive some professional psychotherapeutic support if you feel stuck here. Give yourself the quiet space to listen to what "feeds" you. When you identify those places within you that need care and attention, you can make choices that honor them. We find more moments of presence and deep heart-fullness when we choose activities that line up with our values and needs. More on that in Steps 8 and 9.

Table 1: Values Checklist

Read through the list below, and write a letter next to each value:

V = Very Important, Q = Quite Important, and N = Not So Important.

Try to score at least 10 of them as Very Important.

1. **Acceptance:** to be open to and accepting of myself, others, life, etc. V

2. **Adventure:** to be adventurous; to actively seek, create, or explore novel or stimulating experiences Q

3. **Assertiveness:** to respectfully stand up for my rights and request what I want Q

4. **Authenticity:** to be authentic, genuine, real; to be true to myself V

5. **Beauty:** to appreciate, create, nurture, or cultivate beauty in myself, others, the environment, etc. Q

6. **Caring:** to be caring toward myself, others, the environment, etc. √

7. **Challenge:** to keep challenging myself to grow, learn, improve Q

8. **Compassion:** to act with kindness toward those who are suffering Q

9. **Connection:** to engage fully in whatever I am doing and be fully present with others √

10. **Contribution:** to contribute, help, assist, or make a positive difference to myself or others √ Q

11. **Conformity:** to be respectful and obedient to rules and obligations Q

12. **Cooperation:** to be cooperative and collaborative with others Q

13. **Courage:** to be courageous or brave; to persist in the face of fear, threat, or difficulty Q

14. **Creativity:** to be creative or innovative N

15. **Curiosity:** to be curious, open-minded, and interested; to explore and discover Q

16. **Encouragement:** to encourage and reward behavior that I value in myself or in others √

17. **Equality:** to treat others as equal to myself, and vice-versa Q

18. **Excitement:** to seek, create, and engage in activities that are exciting, stimulating, or thrilling N

19. **Fairness:** to be fair to myself and to others √

20. **Fitness:** to maintain or improve my fitness; to look after my physical and mental health and well-being √

21. **Flexibility:** to adjust and adapt readily to changing circumstances Q

22. **Freedom:** to live freely; to choose how I live and behave, or help others do likewise N

23. **Friendliness:** to be friendly, companionable, or agreeable toward others Q

24. **Forgiveness:** to be forgiving toward myself or to others √

25. **Fun:** to be fun-loving; to seek, create, and engage in fun-filled activities Q

26. **Generosity:** to be generous, sharing, and giving, to myself and to others Q

27. **Gratitude:** to be grateful for and appreciative of the positive aspects of myself, others, and of life in general √

28. **Honesty:** to be honest, truthful, and sincere with myself and others Q

29. **Humor:** to see and appreciate the humorous side of life Q

30. **Humility:** to be humble or modest; to let my achievements speak for themselves Q

31. **Industry:** to be industrious, hard-working, dedicated Q

32. **Independence:** to be self-supportive and choose my own way of doing things Q

33. **Intimacy:** to open up, reveal, and share myself—emotionally or physically—in my close personal relationships Q

34. **Justice:** to uphold justice and fairness N

35. **Kindness:** to be kind, compassionate, considerate, nurturing, or caring toward myself and others √

36. **Love:** to act lovingly or affectionately toward myself or others √

37. **Mindfulness:** to be conscious of, open to, and curious about my here-and-now experience Q

38. **Order:** to be orderly and organized N

39. **Open-mindedness:** to think things through, see things from others' points of view, and weigh evidence fairly Q

40. **Patience:** to wait calmly for what I want N

41. **Persistence:** to continue resolutely, despite problems or difficulties √

42. **Pleasure:** to create and give pleasure to myself or to others N

43. **Power:** to strongly influence or wield authority over others, e.g., taking charge, leading, organizing N

44. **Reciprocity:** to build relationships in which there is a fair balance of giving and taking Q

45. **Respect:** to be respectful toward myself or others; to be polite and considerate, and to show positive regard ✓

46. **Responsibility:** to be responsible and accountable for my actions Q

47. **Romance:** to be romantic; to display and express love or strong affection N

48. **Safety:** to secure, protect, or ensure safety of myself or others Q

⟨6 49. **Self-awareness:** to be aware of my own thoughts, feelings, and actions Y

⟨6 50. **Self-care:** to look after my health and well-being, and get my needs met ✓

51. **Self-development:** to keep growing, advancing, or improving in knowledge, skills, character, and life experience ✓

52. **Self-control:** to act in accordance with my own ideals Q

53. **Sensuality:** to create, explore, and enjoy experiences that stimulate the five senses N

54. **Sexuality:** to explore or express my sexuality N

55. **Spirituality:** to connect with things bigger than myself Q

56. **Skillfulness:** to continually practice and improve my skills, and apply myself fully when using them Q / Y

57. **Supportiveness:** to be supportive, helpful, encouraging, and available to myself or to others ✓ / Q

58. **Trust:** to be trustworthy, loyal, faithful, sincere, and reliable

59. Insert your own unlisted value here:

60. Insert your own unlisted value here:

* * *

Once you've marked each value as V, Q, or N (Very, Quite, or Not So Important), go through all the Vs and select out the top six that are most important to you. Mark each one with a "6," to show it's in your top six. Finally, write those six values out below, to remind yourself this is what you want to stand for as a human being.

Connection	Persistence
Forgiveness	Self-awareness
Gratitude	Self-care

Table 2: Universal Human Needs

Autonomy

Choosing plans for fulfilling one's dreams, goals, values
Liberty
Freedom
Independence
Choice
Individuality
Self-empowerment
Solitude

Celebration of Life

Celebration of the creation of life and dreams fulfilled
Celebration of losses: Loved ones, dreams
Aliveness
Intensity
Stimulation
Excitement
Passion
Pleasure
Delight
Humor
Mourning
Communion

Integrity

Authenticity
Creativity

Dreams
Growth
Meaning
Purpose
Self-respect
Self-worth
Values
Vision

Interdependence

Acceptance
Affection
Appreciation
Being heard/seen
Belonging
Closeness/Intimacy
Communication
Community/Sharing
Cooperation
Connection
Consideration
Contribution to life
Emotional safety/Freedom
Empathy
Equality/Fairness
Friendship/Companionship
Honesty
Love

Predictability/Consistency
Reassurance
Respect
Stability/Reliability
Support
Trust
Understanding

Physical Nurturance
Air
Bonding
Comfort
Nourishment
Movement/Exercise
Physical Affection
Rest
Safety
Sexual Expression
Shelter
Sunlight
Tenderness
Touch
Water

Play
Fun
Laughter
Relaxation

Mental
Stimulation
Clarity
Understanding
Comprehension
Information
Consciousness
Thinking
Reflection
Discrimination

Spiritual Communion
Awareness/Being
Beauty
Giving
Grace
Gratitude
Harmony
Inspiration
Mastery
Order
Peace
Serving

©2017. Excerpted from the work of Marshall Rosenberg, author of *Nonviolent Communication: A Language of Life*

STEP 8

Sustaining Self-Care Practices

If you have time to chatter,
Read books
If you have time to read,
Walk into a mountain, desert, and ocean
If you have time to walk,
Sing songs and dance
If you have time to dance,
Sit quietly, you happy, lucky idiot.

~ Nanao Sakaki

Step 8 is about creating self-sustaining practices. Why do I use this word "practices" instead of "habits" or "routines"? I like the word because it points to the fact that you are trying something new and may need to keep at it for a while for that something new to become a new habit. A wise mentor and

African Healing Dance teacher, Wyoma, introduced me to the concept of establishing daily practices that sustain mind, body, and spirit. Once you get in touch with your values and what nourishes you deeply (Step 7), then you are ready to create activities in your life that reflect those values. When we are doing things we love, we feel more fulfilled—and we are less likely to use food (over-indulgence or restriction) to feel better. Furthermore, creating daily self-care practices helps us to get our needs met by the ideal person to take care of those needs: Ourselves. When we take good care of ourselves, we have more space to reach out and nourish those we love around us. Self-care can be a challenge in busy lives. Sometimes we spend all of our time attending to our work, our children, our friends, our homes, our communities—and all of that is wonderful and rewarding. Care of our Selves often gets squeezed out of the day.

I believe that many of our chronic diseases, our mental illnesses, and our growing fatigues can be boiled down to deficits in self-care. These deficits could be failing to check in with ourselves during the day, appreciating what we are feeling, and knowing when enough is enough. Sometimes we get to the end of the day and realize that we feel depleted. We eat as a reward or a treat—or to give ourselves something good when the day has left us little energy for anything else. Or, conversely, we restrict or obsess about our food intake as a way to feel better about or feel more in control of our lives. We all want lives that are our own, full of joy-filled activities and meaningful moments, even if we are realistic about the inevitable hardships of life at the same time. We do want to learn and grow from our mistakes and challenges in life, but we often punish ourselves instead of seeing the growth in the hardship. **Sometimes we punish ourselves with over- or under-indulgence of food or other pleasures. Why do we do this? We do this because food is tied closely to expressing our larger needs and hungers. It has been so since the time that we cried for our mother's care and feeding on our first day as a human being. Whether we want it to be or not, food will always be associated with love and care and asking for what we need.** Our brains are wired that way from day one on this planet.

We can sometimes be so task-oriented in our lives. We try to cram so many things into a short day or week—even if they are rich, meaningful experiences—that we suffer from a lack of spaciousness. Spaciousness is my favorite self-care practice, and I am the first one to admit that I struggle from lack of it. **Spaciousness** is that luscious time that unfolds naturally in the present moment. In the unfolding, we have room to breathe, to create, to reflect, to have insights, and to make a connection with whomever or whatever is nearby. **I believe that spacious moments encourage creative and spiritual growth spurts.** I grow more deeply connected to my family and friends when we have some lazy, unstructured time together. When I have spacious moments alone, I have insights, notice what's going on inside of me and outside of me, and I notice (when I'm really spacious) that it's all connected. I get clearer about my purpose and feel a sense of clarity and flow. Spaciousness feels very different from the constricted feeling of a deadline; and, yes, if I felt spacious all the time, I'd never get the not-so-fun, deadlined tasks (like finishing this book) done.

Think about a time when you got lost in an activity, which morphed organically into another, and it all seemed to flow together effortlessly. (It's possible, if you are a parent of a young child, that you haven't felt that in some time.) Those "in the flow" afternoons may happen when you are on vacation and have fewer responsibilities, or when you lose track of time on a free afternoon. Whenever they show up, I think you know what I mean. I don't see "spaciousness" in that list of universal human needs, but it's a big one for me. (Perhaps Aliveness, Creativity, Purpose, Harmony, Inspiration, and Peace morph together to create it?) Despite how much I crave spaciousness, I also notice that the active, productive, movement-oriented part of me struggles with unstructured time. I get a little restless. I know that I need a balance of doing, being, and creating, and I am appreciating and trying to listen to this more and more each decade.

I talk with clients often about how those mini-food breaks during the day (you know, the ones where you aren't hungry but find yourself foraging?) may sometimes be the sensory part of us yearning for some downtime. Something rich to eat might give us a five-minute moment of bliss (goddess forbid we stop for more than five minutes!), but is that really what we crave? Perhaps what we really want is the richer taste of spacious time to do or be or make whatever it is that calls to us. We might not feel that we deserve those regenerative moments—but maybe we deserve a bit of chocolate. What would it be like to fill up a little space with whatever calls to us at the moment—with what we really *want* to do, not what we feel *obligated* to do? Perhaps a few minutes to sit meditatively under a tree, or look at the stars, or putter around the house, or write a letter or poem, or maybe even begin to prepare a delicious, health-filled meal. Other things call to us besides food. I have heard my clients and those in my groups talk quite a lot about spiritual food and connection. So many of us hunger for that.

"The grass is always greener where you water it." I can't remember who said this originally. A couple of my clients told me that they think my job is to point out the obvious—which they have somehow forgotten. Yes, when we take good care of ourselves—when we water our grass—it grows. *We grow.* Instead of gazing at our neighbor's green grass (or our neighbor's body, possessions, partner, whatever ...) we can cultivate a greener lawn within ourselves by practicing good self-care. We have to really experiment with how much is enough to know what works for us. Searching out other people's green grass ("She looks so great, so I want to diet like her") won't cut it when you are trying to figure out a way to eat that works specifically for you.

There is no one-size-fits-all eating, exercise, or self-care plan, just like there is no one-size-fits-all amount of work that is right for everyone. Everyone has different thresholds for movement, intimacy, exploration in nature, need for quiet, and need for stimulation. **We are all such wacky, interesting, unique beings, but we often look to others to decide what is best for us. Other people's green grass might be fun to see, certainly; but if we don't play around in our own gardens, then we miss out on the lushness of a fully lived life.**

Some of us are afraid to practice self-care for fear of being seen as selfish or self-serving or self-absorbed. But these are different states than true care of the Self. Self-care fills you up and allows you to be more generous in the world, to give of your unique gifts, and to give without feeling resentful and depleted on the other end. So how do we practice good self-care—when it comes to food or anything else? How do we know when we've eaten enough or the right things for our unique bodies? How do we know how much physical activity is enough to make us feel good and increase our health without taxing our immune systems and making us feel exhausted? How do we really know when enough is enough in our work, relationships, sleep, socializing, or other habits that take time and energy in our lives? Remember when we talked about listening to our own deeper wisdom in Step 4? Discovering our own sustaining self-care practices takes some listening and investigation.

I want to spend a little time on one other non-food way that human beings harm their health: Stress. **Stress affects almost every body system negatively in a chronic state.** (In an acute state, it can make you act to save your life.) Stress alone, in fact, can increase body weight. As I discussed in Step 2 on Body Acceptance, I firmly believe that putting too much attention on weight is counterproductive to healing our relationships with food. But understanding the way stress can affect weight may ease any blame that you place on yourself about where your body is at right now. It also may help you realize that the more you keep toxic and excessive amounts of stress away, the more you decrease your risk for almost all chronic health problems, as well as encourage your body to settle at a weight that is natural for you.

Step 8

Yes, I'm a Health-At-Every-Size dietitian/nutritionist, and I believe there is much more to us than our waistlines. That said, many of my clients struggle with feeling they have more weight on their body than what makes sense, given their lifestyle and history. It feels important to talk about the link between stress and weight—but not so that you feel *compelled* to reduce your stress to lose weight. There's no guarantee of that, and there are many more compelling health and well-being reasons to decrease your stress level. Many of my clients and readers have asked to understand the link between stress and weight, and I think it opens up the possibility for self-compassion to learn about this.

It's no surprise to me that stress plays a role in weight gain. I know that when I have a particularly stressful week, I feel heavier in my body—literally weighed down by the burden of whatever is on my mind. But aside from that general over-whelmed feeling, stress can actually affect our hormonal system in a way that encourages appetite and weight gain. Here's how. Let's say your day at work feels pressured, or your children are pushing every limit all day (or both). Maybe your professor just assigned another paper, and you have two others due already that same week. Maybe your partner just got laid off at the same time a major bill is due. Stress comes in many different forms. And it can also come to us via the internet and TV, as most of the stories in the news today are bleak. Acute stress can initially decrease one's appetite, and this is an adaptive response that primes us for "fight or flight." When they were running from a saber-toothed tiger, it wasn't such a good idea for our ancestors to stop for a snack. However, stressors more chronic than hungry tigers can lead us to eat as a way to soothe ourselves, escape our minds for a moment, or make us feel better in the way that only chocolate can. On top of this emotionally driven increase in eating that some of us experience as a response to stress, there is a genuine hormonal shift that happens in the body that encourages us to keep eating. Here's how it works.

The hormones that are released when we are feeling stressed include adrenaline, corticotrophin-releasing hormone (CRH), and cortisol. High levels of adrenaline and CRH decrease appetite at first, as in the saber-toothed tiger example above, though the effects are not lasting. Cortisol, however, remains elevated in the body long after the initial stress response passes. Elevated cortisol over the long term leads to increased blood-sugar levels. Consistently high blood-sugar levels, along with insulin suppression when the pancreas struggles to keep up with these levels, result in cells starved of glucose. Those cells are crying out for energy, and one way the body regulates this is to send hunger signals to the brain.

Cortisol is also a hormone designed to help you replenish your body after a stressful event has passed, increasing your appetite and driving you to eat more. Again, this works nicely in the case of a saber-toothed tiger. Once we run away and the coast is clear, it's a good idea to nourish ourselves after all that fighting or flighting. But this doesn't really make sense when the tiger is the daily work grind, our partner's messy habits, or Fox News. Typically, we respond to today's stressors not by fighting or flighting (and expending lots of physical energy doing so); we respond by slumping down on the couch, stewing in our anger or frustration, and getting lost in a sports game or Facebook with a large bag of potato chips.

We are much more likely to crave sugar and carbohydrates when we are stressed, as cortisol levels are elevated. If you are stressed, and your body feels soothed and comforted by eating these foods, then you learn something about how to feel better the next time you are stressed. The behavioral pattern becomes established. In this way, eating certain foods resembles an addictive pattern. I say "resembles" because your brain on potato chips in front of Netflix is very different from your brain on crack or alcohol. Some of the psychological connections and brain chemicals are quite similar, though.

Some studies have shown that stress and elevated cortisol increase weight gain not only in general, but also specifically in the abdominal area. Cortisol has a role in fat-cell maturity. If you are in a high-stress, unstable environment, it might make sense to have more "survival fat" around. In this day and age, though, high-stress is less about survival and more about lives that are just too full or pressured. And never mind that your day was so stressful that there was no time for lunch. Add a day of spotty eating to the mix, and you have a recipe for emotional and compulsive eating in the evening. A perfect storm. Your metabolism is slowed down from that spotty amount of food all day; then, the overeating inevitably happens. Some people follow an evening binge with a morning of restricting (or simply not eating much because they are so full from the night before). The cycle continues.

Did I mention that chronic cortisol secretion in the body can constrict blood vessels, increase blood pressure, contribute to gastrointestinal problems, compromise the immune system, and contribute to fertility problems? Whether your urge to over- or under-eat to manage stress is all about hormones or habit (or a little of both), there are things that you can do to disrupt the cycle of stress and cortisol. These changes can benefit your body in many ways. While you have to decide which self-care practices really resonate best for you, I'm going to make a few suggestions that improve cortisol and stress levels. They might be a good place to start.

- **Don't Skip Meals or Go Too Long Without Eating.** Starting the day with breakfast and eating regularly throughout the day will keep blood-sugar levels steady and lower insulin production. Cortisol levels decrease, and you will prevent nighttime overeating.

- **Move Your Body.** The endorphins released by physical activity counteract stress and allow a release of some of that fight-or-flight energy. Most of my clients who feel anxious and/or experience a lot of stress depend on some regular movement or exercise practice to help them manage life. I notice that I get impatient and much less sweet when I'm not able to move to counteract the sitting that I do for my counseling work. Please remember that exercising too hard for too long is actually counter-productive. It can raise cortisol levels and increase stress. Listen to your body, and recognize when you are feeling worn out by your activities. (Injuries, loss of focus after exercise, and needing extra sleep are some indicators.) I often wonder if this is the force at work when my clients work out to exhaustion, seem to eat reasonably well, but find that they are actually gaining weight. Overtraining the body without providing enough calories from food has been shown in research on athletes to decrease lean body mass, increase body fat, and lower resting metabolism. Most active people do not want this outcome. Find an activity that you enjoy. Twenty minutes of walking or yoga counts. When you exercise an appropriate amount, your body releases biochemicals that counter the negative effects of stress hormones and control insulin and blood-sugar levels. I wrote a lot about moving in Step 6. If you want some more inspiration, revisit that chapter.

- **Eat a Balanced, Nutrient-Rich Diet.** Stress has been shown to deplete the body of certain vitamins and minerals, particularly B complex, vitamin C, calcium, and magnesium. These are essential nutrients that balance the effects of cortisol on the body. Eat plenty of vegetables, fruits, and whole grains, as well as foods rich in protein. Step 5 included a lot of information about mindful, balanced eating. Healthful eating keeps stress at bay, too.

- **Sleep Well.** When we don't get enough sleep, cortisol levels rise significantly, which can make us feel hungry all the time. Good sleep also makes it easier for us to avoid a lot of caffeine to keep us going, which then affects our quality of sleep. Reducing caffeine is another way to keep the cortisol/stress cycle at bay.

- **Decrease Caffeine and Alcohol.** Caffeinated coffee and tea, and even chocolate can cause cortisol levels to rise, blood sugar to drop, and hunger to increase. Regular drinking of alcoholic beverages can negatively affect blood sugar and insulin levels, particularly on an empty stomach or in excess.

- **Practice Relaxation.** I say "practice" because many of us have lost the skill of truly relaxing and need to work on it regularly. (Present company included!) We might think that home improvement show is helping us chill out, but the stimulation of the screen and the advertising are actually not calming to our nervous systems. Pure relaxation, in whatever form works for you, produces brain chemicals that counter the effects of stress on the body. Experiment and find out what calms you. Some like sitting and putting their attention on the natural flow of their breath, which is always available. Others find guided or insight meditation, yoga, taking a bath, listening to peaceful music, getting out for a walk in fresh air, or curling up with a good book or a cuddly pet relaxing.

Stress is not inherently evil. It helps us get things done. It creates heroes. But if we feel the effects of stress constantly, especially if we already tend to be on the Type-A spectrum, then it can harm our health and well-being. It weighs us down and keeps us from feeling focused, centered, and present in our lives. As I've said many times before, research shows that so-called weight-loss diets don't work to sustain a long-term healthy weight. Consider the impact that stress might be having on your body and your overall health—and try on a little Type B for a change. On the path to self- and body-love, health, and wellness, finding effective ways to manage stress may be more important than we think.

When we are feeling stress and challenge—which are a part of life—we practice good self-care by coming up with strategies to manage. When we feel anxious after an episode of overeating or a binge, we have a choice. We can beat ourselves up and increase our stress, or we can choose other strategies. We can give ourselves a circular tummy rub (in the direction of digestion: Down and to the right in a spiral around the navel), lie on our left side and rest (also good for digestion), or drink some ginger tea or bubbly ginger brew (good tummy-soothing medicine). We can recognize that we ate in a way that doesn't feel great, suspend judgment about it, and choose to do some self-care practices because we notice that we don't feel good. I guarantee you will learn more from the experience and have a greater chance of making a different choice next time when you treat yourself compassionately and with loving care. I know that's easier said than done when you really feel like beating yourself up for being "bad" again, but promise yourself that you will try to be gentler and more compassionate. You may have to practice this over and over again (like any new habit) before it becomes second nature.

One of my favorite self-care practices is working on being with our thoughts and feelings *as they arise*—noticing them instead of being overtaken by them. The technical term for this technique is **Defusion**, which I learned about in my study of **Acceptance and Commitment Therapy (**ACT**)**, developed by Steven Hayes. I introduced this concept in Step 3, but it bears repeating here. Defusion allows us to not fuse with our thoughts. Try adding, "I'm having the thought that ..." to each negative thought we notice. These additional words help us to observe and not get overly fused with our negative thoughts and feelings. For example, instead of saying, "I'm such a failure—I'll never get this right" and believing it, you can say, "I'm noticing the thought that I'm such a failure and I'll never get this right." Then, you have a little more space to make a self-supporting choice that takes better care of you in that challenging moment. It's subtle, but the regular, many-times-daily dose of this defusion practice has been transformative for many of my clients.

I, too, have a significant inner critic. When I notice what the critic inside of me is saying and label it as an observation—and not "The Truth"—then I step back from the self-defeating stuff my brain likes to throw at me. If you have a huge inner critic that holds you back from taking good care of yourself, I suggest you try the "I'm having the thought that ..." exercise—not just once a day but several. Only then can it be more automatic and help you get unhooked from your negative, self-defeating thoughts. "I'm having the thought that I look fat today." "I'm having the thought that I don't deserve to make myself a good dinner." "I'm noticing that I'm having the thought that I should eat less today." Just because you have the thought doesn't mean you have to do it. Some people with eating disorders like to identify the voice that says, "Don't eat" as their "Eating Disorder Voice." Whatever works for you to separate yourself from those self-defeating thoughts is worth trying!

Beyond negative and self-defeating thoughts is dealing with negative emotions. We all love to feel happiness, joy, excitement, and appreciation. Emotions like anger, sadness, grief, fear, disappointment, and loneliness are less-welcome emotions for most of us; but they are, indeed, part of the human experience and necessary for our growth. For many of my clients, getting used to noticing difficult thoughts and allowing themselves to feel painful feelings is a big part of their healing work. Sometimes the painful feelings are so familiar that we think it's just the way it's going to be. We loop back to sadness, fear, longing, anger repetitively because these feelings had not been met with openness or kindness before. **Meeting feelings with compassion and acceptance—instead of pushing them away—may be a new paradigm, but it can be extremely freeing when practiced.**

For example, try to sit with yourself and your feelings and say, "I hear you. This day was, indeed, a struggle. I'm here with you. We'll get through this." It may sound a little strange at first, but I swear it works! Welcome in your feelings, give them some kindness (especially if you aren't used to being met with gentleness and compassion in your life), and let your feelings unfold. All types of emotions rise to a peak and then fade away. Notice that if you don't *do* something when your anger or sadness is at its peak, but just let it flow, it decreases and eventually goes away (at least until the next time the feeling is triggered). I learned a meditation from Russ Harris, teacher of ACT, called the **Compassionate Hand.** Put a gentle hand on your heart or throat or belly (or wherever you feel an emotion bubbling up), and, over time, you will learn that you have the power to soothe and heal yourself. It may seem strange at first, but it's a practice that can be life-changing when practiced regularly.

Often beginning this work with a trusted therapist helps, particularly when you are out of touch with your body and your emotional pain. If your childhood caregivers who were supposed to be soothing and calming were anything but, then the act of soothing itself can feel somehow toxic or wrong. Self-soothing is a practice, but it can also bring up feelings of feeling unsafe. Negative feelings only get worse if you struggle with them. Trust me on this. If it feels too overwhelming to just *be* with negative emotions, then it is a sign that professional help and support could be valuable.

Let's summarize some of the sustaining self-care practice topics that we visited this chapter—and some additional ones that are on my and my clients' lists of daily or weekly practices:

Eating Patterns That Nourish

Exercise/Movement

Creating Spaciousness

Sleep

Managing Stress

Meditation

Thought Defusion

Pausing Regularly to Check in with Self and Values

Compassionately Sitting with Hard Feelings

Writing/Journaling

Setting Intentions

Being in Nature

Creative Pursuits

Deep Connection with Others

Physical Touch/Hugs/Snuggling

Conscious Breathing

Add any others that help you feel grounded, present, and deeply nourished. You don't have to do this all at once. I recommend picking one or two self-care practices that resonate with you. Once they've become more habitual, choose another. You will be amazed at how much better you feel when you take this time and create intention. When you devote a little more energy to taking good care of yourself—really nourishing your spirit and soul—then the power that food has over you becomes weaker. You may also be able to use psychotherapy, nutrition therapy, and any individual soul work more effectively. I have seen this over and over again. **It's really not all about food. It never was. You heal your relationship with food, body, and self all at the same time by taking good care of *you* in the unique ways that you feel nourished. Take some spacious time to listen deeply, experiment, and discover what you hunger for.**

STEP 9

Developing a
Self-Connected Eating Style

The curious paradox is that when I accept
myself just as I am, then I can change.

~ Carl Rogers

So many of us set goals about weight loss or about change in
diet or exercise. In the United States, gyms get packed and
weight-loss commercials increase around the first of January, the
time of New Year's resolutions. Then, by March (if not before),
the gyms are less crowded. It's as if we forget about our goals until
next January. Then, we feel rather demoralized and ashamed,
as if we have somehow failed or don't have enough willpower or
strength to see our intentions through. Since my primary work is
nutrition therapy, my job is all about assisting in behavior change.
My clients typically want to eat more healthfully, or move more
freely and confidently in their bodies, or discover the freedom

that life without disordered eating can bring. I believe in setting goals (realistic ones) and honoring and being patient with the process to get there. So, how do we look at goals in a new light so that we don't run out of steam weeks or months later?

Each year on my blog, I propose New Year's explorations instead of resolutions. Yes, we want to eat in a way that makes us feel vital and energized, but how do we get to that place? There is nothing wrong with wanting to eat or exercise differently each January—or any time of year—and setting goals to do so. But please don't forget that the reason you might be overindulging in food, drink, or sedentary living could be that you are starving for what matters most to you. You might be trying to fill up or reward yourself with something else. Check in with yourself or your calendar every month during the year to come. Are you filling your life with the things that you most value? If not, I recommend making appointments with yourself to do so. Build that nourishment right into your life the way that you schedule all your other priorities and obligations. Value your needs and desires as much as you value your appointments with others.

Mindful Choices

Punishment and deprivation do not encourage change. (Remember my discussion on dieting in Step 1?) If you want to change a habit, I've found that it works best when you are feeling good about yourself and not when you are beating yourself up. The reality is that we make choices. There is no right or wrong way to eat. But there are consequences for every choice, and there are some decisions that align physically and mentally more with self-care. Sometimes it's having dessert. Sometimes it's not having dessert. When we are feeling connected to our core self and our values (Step 7), we don't have to work so hard to make these choices. Ideally, we choose and let go of the outcome, noticing how we feel and what happens over time. We learn from the choices that we make. We can opt to eat the light and fresh salad greens, or the more grounding sandwich, or the ice cream cone because it's a hot summer day and that's what we feel like having. We can choose the entree that speaks to our palates—and seems interesting and aligned with our values and preferences—without second-guessing ourselves.

Ideally, we slow down and savor every bite because the food is delicious and worth enjoying. We aren't eating a certain amount of calories or carbs or points. Instead, we are eating life-giving, pleasure-providing food. We will eat just enough of it because we are staying present with the eating experience, paying enough attention to the food and our bodies as we eat it. We take in the sensory enjoyment of the food, the texture, the warmth or coolness, the flavors, the feelings of hunger and satiety. We are in our bodies when we eat—not in our heads. It's not that we don't use our minds or our knowledge about nutrition to make decisions about eating when we eat intuitively. An obvious example is, "Eating that full bag of Cheetos last time made me feel sick. I don't want to do that again." Here you are using your mind and your experience to make a wise food choice, not just your body's current state. When you see your body as a living, breathing miracle, and focus on nurturing and caring for it with life-giving, healthful food, there is a very different focus. There is no deprivation. There are no "shoulds" or "shouldn'ts," only certain foods that feel better to your body than others. There are no mistakes—only opportunities to learn what foods feel best. There is (ideally) no criticism and guilt. Again, there are just choices.

Does this natural, body-centered way of eating seem like pie in the sky? It just might involve reprogramming everything that you learned about food as you grew up, bringing you back to how you ate when you were a toddler. Back then, you knew that a few bites of a cookie were enough when there were other pleasures in life to explore. If it feels foreign to go back to this way of eating, you might appreciate some coaching and support along the way. Once practiced regularly, mindful, intuitive eating is liberating, and brings you into your healthiest body. That body might not be the "ideal body" that you envision, but it will be a respected, honored, and well-nourished one. And isn't that what is important? It's not how we look in that bikini, really; it's the fact that we are out enjoying the sunshine. Don't let anyone—the diet industry, well-meaning relatives, your partner, your inner critic—tell you that you should look different. (If they do, it may be because they have their own body-image insecurities, and they are projecting them onto you.)

Don't let anyone trick you into thinking that your body size and shape are more important than feeding yourself in a way that aligns with your own body's needs. And, please don't let any nutrition and health guru tell you what's best for you to eat. My colleagues in nutrition often commiserate about being stalked in the grocery store. Someone even followed one of my dietitian friends around a buffet table, saying that she was going to take exactly what my friend was putting on her plate. Don't think for a moment that we nutritionists somehow have the answers to what *all* bodies should have to eat at any given moment. We don't!

One day, as I was writing this chapter, I noticed a little hunger. It was about an hour and a half before I was to meet a friend for some lunch together. I wanted to enjoy the treat of eating lunch out for a change (instead of my usual leftovers from the night before). I noticed, though, that I was hungry enough that I was getting a little distracted from my work. I remembered that my breakfast of homemade pancakes with my kids had less protein than my usual egg breakfast, which typically holds me until lunch. (I can't help thinking like this as a nutritionist.) I reached inside my office snack drawer and pulled out a few handfuls of nut-heavy trail mix. The bits of chocolate chips inside were a satisfying pick-me-up along with the nuts, and I knew this would hold me over the next couple of hours until lunch. All of this decision-making took a few minutes (probably not as much time as it took for me to type and edit this paragraph), but it's a demonstration of how intuitive, mindful eating helped me to feel good as I went along in my day. Obviously, I had to have the practice of keeping ready-to-eat snacks that work for me nearby. This pattern of snacking at 11:00 a.m. is not one I usually follow, nor is it a prescription of any sort—but, on this day, I took good care of myself and increased my late-morning productivity at work by honoring the message that my body was giving me.

Karen Koenig, the author of *Starting Monday*, writes that Trial and Error means trying different foods and noticing what tastes and feels good. Trial and Error takes some time and attention. It means cultivating trust in yourself by having an idea and not being too afraid to test it out and see how it feels, even if it's something that no one else around you considered. Again, you can notice that green grass of your neighbor, but please don't forget to water and care for your very own garden. Just a few examples of what you might come up with as you apply Trial and Error to self-care are:

- I need to have a substantial breakfast to have balanced eating the rest of the day.

- I need at least seven hours of sleep to feel focused and alert.

- Working out four times per week is just right for me.

- Getting together with friends in person a couple of times per week helps me feel connected.

Create your own set of practices around what you need to feel balanced (Step 8) and test them out by setting manageable, measurable goals. Notice the numbers in the above examples. That's the measurable part. How do you feel when you try this out? Was your goal too much, too little, or just enough?

Enoughness

Practice listening to your own, personal sense of "enoughness" in your life. Just because everyone in your office works fifty-plus hours each week doesn't mean that this lifestyle is healthiest for you. As you pay attention to your own needs and limits and gradually learn to trust yourself more, you will develop the ability to take good care of yourself. Karen Koenig writes, again in her book *Starting Monday*, "Trust produces confidence, which produces more trust, and each reinforces the other."

Practice listening to your sense of enoughness with food each day. Notice that sometimes a whole sandwich is just right, sometimes a half. See what types of food make your body and mind feel good. I find this work on "enough" is one of the last frontiers of eating-disorders recovery, and it's often something that has to be revisited even by those of us who are quite far along in recovery. It comes up around other things when you no longer use food as a way to deal with challenges. **Through the process of recovering from disordered eating, your sense of being enough, doing enough, and saying, "Enough is enough" generally gets easier over time. At a certain point in the recovery process, we stop choosing to eat (or starve) to make us feel better. Instead, we ask for what we need and soothe our own emotions. By directly honoring our needs and feelings, we learn how to take good care of ourselves.**

Jessica walked into her session saying that she imagined herself lying face down on the rug in my office, pounding her fists. I told her that she was certainly welcome to embody her feelings. Although she chose not to hit the floor, she did cry more forcefully than usual this session. Jessica has been feeling very frustrated with her eating. She had been eating lots of things that she considers "non-food," like Cheez-Its. Jessica has been preparing and cooking "real" food she considers healthy, but then she chooses not to eat it while at work, going out to get other, "less healthy" takeout food. The other day she ended up eating a whole pizza.

Her tears came with feelings of hopelessness: "I am not strong enough to do what I need to do to take care of my health, and I'm going to kill myself with my bad habits." I tried to reframe this for her. Could she observe her eating habits less judgmentally, so that she has more room to problem-solve? For example, on Monday she was exhausted from all the housecleaning she'd done over the weekend. Instead of beating herself up and saying that she can't get her eating right, I invited her to use curiosity. She came up with a much-less-critical assessment of her eating. It went something like this: "Hmmm ... I am really exhausted this Monday after the weekend. Weekends are supposed to be my rest from work. Something is not working for me. I know I treated myself to that food partly because I wanted to take care of myself in some way or soothe myself because I was exhausted. Maybe I need more help, or to lower my standards about cleaning on the weekend, or something else ..."

Jessica's work in high-tech is stressful and demanding—and the standard in her industry is perfection-or-you-may-lose-your-job. Perfectionism contributed to her negative self-talk, too. She ate something that didn't feel "right" for her to eat. In her own view, she'd failed at taking care of herself, even though she had just been doing her best to cope with her circumstances. Binge-eating may have consequences that don't feel so good, but it's a very effective coping strategy that many of us use when we want soothing. We also often use food when we want to get out of our heads and into our bodies to experience some sensory pleasure for a short time.

Jessica wants to eat a vegan, plant-based, very low-fat diet, but she can't seem to do it. Eating food that tastes good is also important to her. This "hyper-clean" way of eating ends up feeling like a diet, and it doesn't leave her fully satisfied. When she feels deprived, she rebels and seeks out highly palatable foods that fill her up. The cycle starts again when she feels guilty about eating in an "unclean" way, and she goes back to her "virtuous" eating. The overeating-and-regaining-control-and-overeating cycle continues.

I suggested that when Jessica experiences a craving or a desire for cheese, she think about a way that she can honor her craving for cheese and still create a healthy meal with it. Instead of being black-and-white (she either won't eat cheese at all, or she will eat a whole cheese pizza), she could have a sandwich with hummus and tomatoes and melted cheese. To her, this sounded yummy and health-giving. The part of her that is rigidly clinging to the strict vegan plan will not see this as healthy, but it is still a better choice for her body than the large cheese pizza that ends up making her feel very sick afterward. Jessica thought she could try this concept of listening to—instead of denying—her cravings and working with them to find a balanced food choice. (This is not to say, by the way, that pizza is not a viable option, too. For Jessica, however, this was not the kind of meal that she really wanted to eat in the middle of her workday, and it didn't feel good in her particular body.)

I suspected that Jessica would struggle with finding this balance, as gray is always more of a challenge for her (and many of us!) than black-and-white. I also suspected that while her work and home life feel so stressful and she's not getting enough sleep, it will be hard for her to take care of herself with food and find this balance. She admits that she uses her struggles around food as a way to avoid more difficult things and to feel like she has some control over her life. I love the way Jessica called her binge-eating "lubrication," something that helps her through tough times. She also acknowledged that it is lubrication with "grit" in it—consequences that make it less helpful to her body, mind, and spirit. By seeing her binge-eating and restriction cycle as a coping strategy, she could invite a little more compassion toward herself into this process.

Since the session in which she wanted to pound her fists into my floor, Jessica has been gradually embracing the "middle road" in her eating. She is not eating in the most virtuous way that she has always wanted to eat, but she tried it for decades, and it didn't work. Jessica is starting to let it go. As a result, she is not doing as much binge-eating—particularly when she is being mindful and present and slows down enough to make her self-care a priority. It's been quite a journey, and I am honored to be a supportive witness to her growth and determination as she improves her relationship with food.

Vegetarianism and Plant-Based Eating

I think it's worth spending a little time on the questions many of my clients bring in about different ways to eat. A common dilemma for some is whether or not to adopt plant-based or vegetarian eating. In my practice, I do not prescribe either across the board; instead I assist clients in deciding if these are styles of eating they wish to explore. A lot of information exists out there about plant-based eating and its benefits in preventing chronic disease, maintaining overall health, and supporting the environment. In Step 7, we learned about how our values might impact our eating style—as well as how clarifying values can help solidify body acceptance and decrease an obsession with eating flawlessly. Eating style, in my mind, is ideally a composite of preferences, values (including orientation toward health), and lifestyle.

I do not believe in a one-size-fits-all approach to eating. I also do not believe that all individuals need to orient their eating and other lifestyle choices toward health. Judging someone else's diet as more or less healthy is not my role as a nutritionist. For those who want to orient themselves toward health and well-being, I can assist them in making decisions, but I never assume that all people value health the same way. In fact, there are lots of things in life worth appreciating; health and well-being are only two of them.

Vegetarianism suits some people and aligns with their values. Sometimes people wish to eat vegetarian, but when they try it out, they discover it doesn't work for their particular body and lifestyle. If a plant-based diet connects with your values and health goals, then there are lots of ways to "do" it. Instead of feeling you did something wrong when you ate outside your values, the goal is to make conscious choices. If you chose to eat meat when you want to eat mainly a vegetarian diet, then do be kind to yourself and admit you made a choice. Notice how you feel afterwards—in body and mind—and use that information to assist you with further decisions. **I recommend** dispensing with food rules and swapping them for choices. Notice which choices feel right and which choices don't. I firmly believe that is the best way to embody your eating and eat well for your unique self.

When I got pregnant with my now-twelve-year-old twins, I was mostly a plant eater, though not a strict vegetarian. I never really liked most meats when I was a kid, always hiding the meat in many of my meat-and-potatoes dinners (often drowning it in ketchup). Although I ate some meat regularly pre-pregnancy, I never really craved it. I was always more inclined toward the vegetarian or seafood choice on a menu. However, once I was pregnant, I was astounded by how much I craved meat. I'd never experienced this before. Since I was a nutritionist, I interpreted these cravings as my body really asking for more protein and iron for the development of my babies. Sometimes I was so hungry that I felt like I could eat a whole chicken! I was never a huge fan of mayonnaise before pregnancy, but I craved and ate a lot of chicken salad when I was pregnant. I'm sure I must have needed all that protein and fat.

I trusted my body and listened to how much I needed to eat, gained a lot of necessary weight, and gave birth to healthy, full-term twins. I can't take full credit for the outcome of my pregnancy, as there are so many factors involved in growing babies; but I believe that listening to my body and what it wanted during that time was an important act of self- (and child) care. I honed my body-listening during this period since my body seemed to be even more clear about what it wanted and what it didn't want. I have heard this over and over again from pregnant moms. There is a desire to take good care of the body during this time, but there also seems to be clearer signals from the body about what that care might be.

To Gluten or Not to Gluten?

It's probably no surprise that I'm not a fan of the many new diets that eliminate or reduce major food groups. Currently, the food criminals are flour, sugar, gluten, or carbohydrates in general. Now, some people do indeed have gluten intolerance, wheat allergies, or celiac disease and need to avoid some forms of carbohydrate for their health and well-being. However, there are more and more people dramatically reducing carbs with the goal of weight loss, vitality, or world peace. There is no question that many people in the Western world eat more grain-based and sugary foods than their bodies might need. However, the recent fad to lower carbohydrates across the board is reminiscent of the low-fat, no-fat craze in the '80s and '90s, which was going strong when I started my work in nutrition. (If you are as old as I am, you might remember Snackwell Cookies. They were fat-free, and we somehow felt like we could eat whole sleeves of them, even though they replaced all the fat with sugar.) I have an old nutrition-practice handout from that time about the many benefits of fat in our diet that I just never use anymore. Most people aren't afraid of eating fat these days.

Today it has become rather mainstream to give up gluten or dairy or sugar or meat or soy or all of the above. While I will never argue against eating more fruits and vegetables, I am concerned about the way in which certain styles of eating are making some of us feel more virtuous than others. I am concerned about how badly we are made to feel when we aren't able to stick to a more "virtuous" way to eat.

There are many people in my practice and in my social circles (myself included) who have food allergies and sensitivities, so I appreciate the way certain foods can make us feel better or worse—or even quite sick. **Celiac disease**, for example, is a genuine condition in which it is quite dangerous to be eating foods that contain gluten. Gluten is a mixture of two proteins that are found in cereal grains, particularly wheat, and it gives dough its elastic texture. Someone with celiac disease can now find restaurants and stores with items that meet their dietary restrictions. I appreciate the fact that food allergies are being taken seriously—as many of them are life-threatening. More ingredients lists are available for customers who truly need them.

Food allergies or sensitivities mostly show up as symptoms of the lungs, throat, sinuses, skin, or joints. They can also have behavioral consequences, like irritability, which are harder to pinpoint. **Food intolerances** are different from allergies. Intolerances tend to create digestive symptoms like bloating, gas, or diarrhea. The most common one is lactose intolerance, a problem digesting the carbohydrate portion of milk. Lactose intolerance is different from a milk or dairy allergy, which is most often an allergy to the protein part of the milk, called casein.

Gluten sensitivity is not celiac disease, but there is evidence that it is a real condition. Some people are, indeed, less able to tolerate gluten and will feel better if they don't include foods with gluten in their diets. When you do a food elimination for a short time, and then the foods with gluten are added back, you will notice symptoms if you are sensitive. A client who is gluten sensitive swears that when she eats gluten, she feels like "her emotions have *her* instead of her having her emotions." Who am I to disprove this experience? I always recommend that, if you think you might be sensitive to gluten, you get the blood test for celiac disease first. (You have to be eating gluten, though, for the test results to be correct.) That way, you know if your gluten sensitivity could lead to more serious, life-threatening problems if you don't fully eliminate this food component. People with celiac disease ideally shouldn't even nibble on wheat bread or use cutting boards that were used to slice it. It's that dangerous for someone with celiac disease to eat gluten, so being clear about what kind of intolerance you have is important.

Food sensitivities and intolerances are harder to identify than allergies, and many clients come in wondering if they have some. Again, the best way to pinpoint whether or not you are sensitive to a particular food is to eliminate the one food (even little amounts of it) for four to six weeks. After that time, reintroduce the food, monitoring for any symptoms. If you end up eating the food accidentally during that period, you have to start the elimination period again. Skin symptoms, for example, don't show up right away. Getting the food out of your system takes time. I find that doing this elimination one food at a time helps with compliance to the removal and decreases the feelings of deprivation that come from taking away food that you may enjoy. Only you can determine if you feel better on or off certain foods. I encourage elimination trials very, very cautiously in my practice. **I recommend that clients work on their relationship with food and any emotional issues that lead to under-eating, overeating, or chaotic eating before they try** *any* **food-elimination protocol.** Symptoms that might be relieved by eliminating food may also go away by eating in a more intuitive, body-connected way, especially digestive symptoms. It's hard to tease out the results of the elimination trial if, going into the trial, your eating is also feeling out of whack as a whole. If you have an eating disorder—or active symptoms of disordered eating—I firmly believe that working on normalizing your eating patterns is the priority. Only then, with a more balanced relationship with food, are you ready to try a food elimination to see if it will improve any lingering symptoms or discomfort.

If you are wondering if it would help you feel better to eliminate some food or food group, go deep inside yourself, and ask yourself the following questions:

- **Do I want to remove this food because I truly believe that I will feel better in my body if I don't eat it—and not just because I want to feel more in control of my eating, or my body, or my life?**

- **Do I want to eliminate a particular food to see if my health improves—and not for weight loss?**

- **Am I willing to try eliminating this food for about four to six weeks (and is it safe and feasible for me to do so) and then adding it back to notice the changes in my symptoms?**

If you answered "Yes" to these questions, then you might be ready to entertain the idea of testing yourself for a food sensitivity. But first, ask the next two questions:

- **Am I frequently under-eating, overeating, or eating erratically (going long times without eating much food and then eating a lot all at once)?**

- **Do I frequently eat emotionally, so that my emotions, thoughts, and stress may be affecting the way I feel when I eat food as much or more than the actual foods that I eat?**

If you answered "Yes" or even "Maybe" to one or both of these questions, then I recommend putting your energy into finding more balance in your life and eating patterns before investigating food sensitivities. Erratic eating is very often the culprit when it comes to gastrointestinal symptoms. Also, we *all* eat emotionally sometimes; but if you do so often, then working on your relationship with food and your body may be more valuable up front than finding out if you have a gluten sensitivity.

Other Food Allergies/Sensitivities

About two-thirds of people have a hard time digesting cow's milk. Some people are intolerant of the carbohydrate portion of the milk (lactose) and have digestive symptoms. Some people are intolerant of the protein portion of the milk (casein) and have lung/sinus/skin symptoms. Some have both. With lactose intolerance, symptoms can vary from person to person. In other words, someone might have no symptoms with yogurt, because the cultures added to yogurt help to break down the lactose and make it easier to digest, but then have major symptoms (diarrhea and bloating) after drinking milk. Some people's lactose intolerance is mild, and they can eat all kinds of dairy products as long as they don't have more than, say, two in one day.

When I discovered my daughter's cow's milk sensitivity, I noticed skin and sinus changes that completely disappeared when she stopped eating dairy products for a while. We kept allowing small amounts of cow's milk in baked goods and butter here and there, giving her body a chance to build up a tolerance slowly. She started to add back a little cheese without consequence and, at this point, seems to have grown out of her allergy. She no longer has any symptoms when she eats dairy products, though she has never developed a taste for straight cow's milk. Food allergies may be outgrown, particularly in children. The wisdom today is that the food not be entirely eliminated (unless there is a life-threatening anaphylactic reaction). Small amounts of butter and milk (such as in baked products) given to a child with a cow's milk allergy, for example, will keep the child exposed to tiny amounts of the allergen.

This tolerance-building can happen—sometimes with less success—in adults, too. You might eliminate an irritating food for a time, and once your symptoms have improved, you can add it back to your diet without consequence. If that happens, it's likely that the food sensitivity was related to your gut health. Some rest and repair could make it possible for you to eat that food again. Describing this process is outside the scope of this book. I recommend checking out my colleague

Nicole Spear's book *Healthy Gut, Healthy Life* if you'd like to learn more and, again, when your relationship with food feels more solid.

What I find most worrisome is the way that so many people today avoid certain food categories without actually testing the reality in their own bodies. They just believe that because some celebrity feels good off dairy, they must, too. I also worry when someone thinks that taking away certain foods is going to be the answer to their challenging relationship with food. For example, they believe that by eliminating sugar, flour, and gluten, they will halt their compulsive eating. I rarely find this to be true, even though I strive to work with my clients' food preferences as they heal from whatever pain and suffering underlie the drive to cope using food. Most of the time, cutting out certain food groups just feels like another diet and creates that deprivation mindset. And, by now, I hope I've convinced you that most diets fail to be sustainable.

A registered dietitian or nutrition therapist who has expertise in disordered and emotional eating may be able to help you find some balance in your diet and help you decide if decreasing certain foods might make you feel better. Beware of any nutrition professional who tries to give you a prescriptive way of eating or tells you to eliminate some foods that you don't have a self-tested allergy or sensitivity to. Find a nutrition therapist who is interested in your relationship with food and your body and will tease out any of those issues *first*, before doing a food-sensitivity challenge. My clients often hear me say that there is a difference (and it can be a fine line) between not eating something because it aligns with your values not to eat it, and not eating something because it aligns with an eating disorder—or a desire for control over your body and weight.

Food Addiction?

I acknowledge the addictive quality inherent in some foods in our food supply, but there is more work to healing an addiction than just eliminating the addictive substance. Sometimes a client will cut out sugar, believing that it will make her feel more in control of her food choices or her life. Often, at first, that is how it feels; but generally, the real reasons that her eating or her life seems out of control still exist. Instead of admitting that sugar-free was not the answer to her deeper life challenges, she feels like a failure. I also find that, when someone tries to cut out lots of carbohydrate foods, he often ends up craving these foods that are vital to health.

Food can create a dopamine response in the brain, which fuels a psychologically-based attraction to the food. While the addictive quality of eating is magnitudes different than the addictive quality of alcohol, drugs, or other substances, we can use food to numb, escape, and soothe the way other substances get used. For some, binges take on a life of their own. The binge-eaters feel like addicts, powerless against the food. I can honestly say that, in my decades of work with compulsive eaters (and my own history), feeling helpless keeps the cycle of compulsive eating going. But making choices from a place of agency and belief in recovery heals. The changes may need to be small, but they build on each other. **Food is not something that we can avoid, like alcohol or crack. We deal with food several** times per day in order to live. **Abstinence with compulsive eating, in my belief, does not at all work the same way as abstinence with other non-vital substances. We have to have a relationship with food.** I have seen people disappointed by this over and over and over again. I will own my bias here, but it's an inclination based on much anecdotal evidence—not only my own, but those of many of my esteemed colleagues who also work to assist people in breaking free of compulsive eating.

I often talk to my clients about "finding the gray" when it comes to food, since many are used to thinking in very black-and-white terms. They see foods as good or bad, virtuous or decadent, on their list or off of it. The idea that there are no wrong foods, just more or less health-giving ways of eating, is a hard concept to digest. In fact, what feels like a health-giving way to eat for one person may not work for another. Look around and observe all the diverse body types out there. I just won't believe that all those unique bodies need the same kinds of food all the time! **I believe that we are what we eat, in a sense, but I also believe that our bodies are quite resilient. When we listen within to our own internal wisdom about what to eat (and how much of it) at any given moment, a beautiful, trusting relationship with our bodies—and eventually with food—develops. But this process requires letting go of "rules" and being comfortable with gray.**

Let's think for a moment about the softness of the color gray. I happen to like this color, but it's not just because I'm discovering more of it on my head as I approach fifty. I like gray because it is not too perfectly clean or rigid, like black or white. It's flexible and shifting, like fog, which means it requires a leap of faith to perceive what is behind it. Think fluffy clouds or soft gray animal fur or smooth stones at the beach. Embrace the not-so-perfect weather, the softness, the unknowing. Once your thinking allows for more gray, there are more possibilities, and you just might not want to go back to black-and-white again.

My client Janet talked about the part of her that feels like an impulsive young child when she binge-eats sugary foods. Although some people may find that avoiding the substance that they crave (like sugar) works for them, most people discover that avoidance is unsustainable. Janet's work is about caring for that impulsive young child within and giving her some of the limits that perhaps were not given to her in a secure, loving way when she was a child. I encourage clients to work toward an inner impulse control that is neither rigid and authoritarian nor overly permissive and self-destructive. Gray, again. Somewhere between the no-sugar-ever and the eat-whatever-I-want-whenever-I-want-to is this inner parent-like force of loving, self-care that says, "You may have a piece of chocolate, but after you first give your body a nutritious snack," or "You may go into the candy store, but spend only two dollars."

"Spot-Clean" Eating

Today everyone is talking a lot about "Clean Eating." I'm all for a let's-get-back-to-recognizing-our-food way of life. I appreciate shorter ingredients lists—ones where I can find whole foods listed and not chemicals. I like shopping at farmers' markets, eating seasonally and locally. I believe in all of this, and I believe that our bodies and the planet benefit when we eat more whole food and more plants. But as a nutrition therapist and eating-disorders specialist, I worry about us taking clean eating too far. Now, you might say, isn't it clear that some foods are really more healthful than others? Remember, I'm not talking about unconscious eating here. I truly believe that when we make conscious choices, thinking about our own innate preferences as well as what foods feel best in our bodies (this sometimes takes trial and error), we end up eating in a balanced, healthy way most of the time. So many of my clients have "shoulds" that get in the way of actually tuning in to what feels best in their bodies. Sometimes the foods they say they "shouldn't" eat become more attractive just because they are forbidden.

That's why I am consistently bothered by the flurry of conflicting nutritional advice on the internet. How can someone who doesn't know my body and lifestyle tell me how to eat? Personally, I learned over many years the kinds of meals and snacks that "work" for me. And, in the process, I have maintained enough flexibility so that I can enjoy so many different kinds of foods in different settings. Every once in a while, I discover something that doesn't feel great in my body. I had some hot peppered oil recently that didn't sit well with me (though my go-to ginger remedy helped my stomach feel better). I now know that if I go to that particular restaurant again, I'll go lighter on the hot pepper oil. I learned from my body's experience. If I trust the latest advice from a nutritional guru on the internet, I might bypass the wisdom that my own body affords me every time I pay attention when I eat. If I set up a "should eat" situation (that the rebellious part of me might want to undo), then I decide what to eat away from my own values and preferences regarding food. The eating experience is bound to be less satisfying when I apply "shoulds" than if I am making choices from my own body wisdom, learning, and self-care.

Elizabeth has been working hard on finding gray areas in her life. She has operated from all-or-nothing, black-or-white decisions in many ways. She recently talked about an instance where she found the gray regarding housecleaning. Bear with me, as it's a strange example, but it works. Long ago, my client read in a housekeeping magazine that she was supposed to wash her bathroom floors weekly. She has had that task on her (extensive) to-do list for a long time but realized that it was often not getting done. And she was really beating herself up about it, particularly when time would go by and she really didn't like the way the floors looked. It was black-or-white thinking that kept her stuck. She either cleaned the bathroom entirely, moving all the furnishings and making the floors gleam—or she let it go and had to live with floors that were messier than she liked. It never occurred to her—until last week—that she could spot-clean the floors in between. Instead of thorough weekly cleaning, she could clean the floors really well monthly and then spot-clean in between (picking up the hair and other things that collect on the bathroom floor without the whole procedure).

So, what does this have to do with food? I think it parallels some of her struggles with eating. Elizabeth also goes back and forth between eating "perfectly" and "cleanly"—following all of the rules of the blogs and websites that she follows—or she rebels and starts eating, in her words, "… like crap." She knows that neither feels good, although the "cleaner" eating has the illusion of feeling great at first; it's just never been sustainable.

So, we had a good laugh together when we considered that she could "spot-clean" her eating, too. Just like the spot-cleaning of her bathroom made her squirm at first (imagining all those germs and gross things under her furnishings), eating in this more middle way is hard to get used to. But, just like the spot-cleaning of her house gave her more freedom and rest to pursue other passions, the spot-clean eating (versus the perfect and unsustainable clean eating) set her free and shifted her challenging relationship with food. Instead of eating a large plate of just vegetables or a whole box of plain buttered pasta (one virtuous, in her mind, and one not), she can combine the vegetables and noodles and make a middle-of-the-extremes dish that is satisfying and feels good in her body.

So, the next time you are out and about and you don't know if the yummy meal your friends are serving you is as "clean" as the version that you eat at home ... Please don't panic, don't starve, don't ruminate over the ingredients! Make an informed choice whether to eat it or not, based on your own knowledge of what feels good in your body and your own values. When you find yourself frustrated with eating "good" and "bad" interchangeably, try to give up the struggle and stop judging yourself and your eating. I propose Spot-Clean eating versus Clean Eating, which allows flexibility, pleasure, ease, and space for the rest of the joys of living.

A Word About Food, Mood, and Gut Health

All bodies are different and they respond to foods differently. In fact, our mood can affect how we respond to food, too. If you've ever had a stomachache before a major interview, do you blame the food you just ate, or do you blame the stress about the interview? Sometimes it's both. Certain foods "mix" better with stress than others. (Yes, comfort foods sometimes really are soothing.) Sometimes we aren't even aware that we are stressed or anxious or keyed up about something. We sometimes blame the food we ate, but it may simply be that the stress constricted, slowed down, and aggravated our digestion.

Today there is so much information about gastrointestinal (GI) health and wellness than ever before. The field of GI nutrition is exploding, and even I can barely keep up with the new developments in the study of the microbiome. While it's outside of the scope of this book to address all GI issues here, I find in my practice that resolving conditions like constipation, diarrhea, irritable bowel syndrome, indigestion, colitis, and reflux can go a long way toward helping you heal your relationship with food—and your body. Often, when clients eat more regularly and in a more balanced way, incorporating many of the principles outlined in these Steps, their irritable bowel, indigestion, or constipation improves or goes away entirely. Sometimes more aggressive measures, medications, or supplements may be needed—particularly if the GI conditions have gone on for a long time. I recommend seeking out the help of a registered dietitian, functional medicine nutritionist, gastroenterologist, or other practitioner specializing in gut health to assist in this area if your symptoms are severe or impeding your ability to work on these 10 Steps.

Self-Compassion and Goal-Setting

Kristin Neff, the author of the book *Self-Compassion*, wrote, "So why is self-compassion a more effective motivator than self-criticism? *Because its driving force is love, not fear.*" Love makes us feel secure and confident as we raise our feel-good oxytocin levels in the body. Fear makes us feel insecure and anxious as cortisol—which I addressed back in Step 8—gets released in our bodies. Kristin Neff writes that instead of asking if you're good enough (self-criticism), self-compassion asks, "What's good for you?" If you care for yourself, you'll want to do what you need to do to learn, grow, and create habits that express that self-love. You will eat in a way that sustains you and makes you feel good, even if that means you sometimes have to say "No" to something that you like. Any good parent will sometimes say "No" to a child's wishes, out of love and caring. We do the same for ourselves, with conviction and with ease, when we love and care for ourselves.

If you make a food choice that doesn't feel good or hurts you or your health in some way, I invite you to say compassionately, "I'm sorry. That didn't feel right, did it? Well, now I've learned something that I can use the next time I'm in that food situation." Do you feel how kind and patient that sounds? Is this what you say to yourself when you polish off a pint of ice cream and feel sick? Is that how you address yourself when you restrictively eat all day, only to find yourself picking late at night on all the things you forbade during the day? I assure you that kindness and curiosity—instead of criticism—will go a long way toward creating habits that help you feel cared for and that are sustainable.

I firmly believe that on our path toward wellness, the more we eat with presence and mindfulness and listen to our bodies, the more we find that our bodies can handle a wide variety of foods. We usually find that we enjoy most foods prepared with love, care, and attention. If you believe that not incorporating a particular food into your diet will help you feel better, then do so in a way that listens to your body and what it has to say. Please don't give up gluten or flour or sugar or meat because it's fashionable in certain circles to say that you do. Be your own investigative reporter. Take small, measurable steps to change any eating habits that don't make you feel your best. Try one or two changes per week, ideally things that are about a "3" or "4" on a scale of "0 to 10" in difficulty. Over time, the changes that are an "8 or more" will likely move down the list and seem less daunting.

I really encourage you to start with baby steps. Agreeing with yourself to incorporate one new vegetable per week may be more realistic than trying for five a day. Trying to add back in a favorite sweet food that you once forbade (so that it's not so charged and fraught with guilt) is also best done gradually and with consciousness. Aiming to stop counting calories, when you've done so for years, might be tricky. Perhaps seeking to buy one new food this week—without looking at the calorie content—is the best way to slowly break down the obsession into manageable steps.

I wish that I could say that diving in and changing everything about your eating and self-care habits at once works. It does for some. I have a friend who successfully changed his food almost overnight when he got his diabetes diagnosis. It was a big motivator. But he'd never had a particularly challenging relationship with food or his body. I find those of us who have struggled with food for a while succeed at healing in small steps that continually build.

It's hard to listen to your body if you typically eat for external versus internal reasons. You will eventually find that food is more enjoyable when you intrinsically choose it. I will like the meal more because it's what I really feel like eating in the moment and not because it's the healthiest option based on this week's "top ten health foods." Be patient if tuning in to your body is hard. Be patient if you can't locate what it is that you feel like eating. Make your best guess. And then actually listen to how it feels. You might discover that eating a few pieces of bread before the main dish leaves you feeling full and not really interested in eating the yummy meal. You might non-judgmentally notice that this doesn't feel good, and make the decision to save some of your appetite for the meal by eating less of the bread. This is very different than making a rule that says "no bread." The quality of making choices and learning from those choices—when they work out well and when they don't—creates freedom in eating that is very different from eating according to outside rules.

I recently discovered that eating my favorite Thai food at 10:00 p.m. didn't feel so good the next day. I typically like how that food nourishes my body—but not so close to bedtime. I made a mental note that my favorite dish, even eaten mind-fully—and according to my appetite, where I didn't end up finishing the whole dish—didn't feel so good in my body so close to sleep. This is very different from setting a rule for myself that says I can't eat anything after 9:00 p.m. I eat food at all times of the night if I'm hungry without the same consequence, but that spicy, heavy Thai food that I love just doesn't work for me so late. I suspect I won't have a craving for it, in the same way, the next time I work a late night. That bit of listening to my body reminded me to eat a more substantial dinner earlier in the evening on the nights when I will be up late writing.

I'm constantly learning about what works for me around food and what doesn't. I'm not setting up rules (that I will eventually break), but noticing my preferences and what feels great in my body. In fact, I didn't think about the Thai food experience so much until I decided to tell it as an example in this book. These days I make food choices based on what historically has felt good to me and what feels good to eat at the moment. I base this on my proximity to food, so I keep foods that I know I love around me. (And, fortunately, after a long day of work, certain Thai restaurants stay open late when my desire for a grounding, comforting dish of warm food strikes.)

I didn't always eat this way. I developed a lot of "shoulds" and "shouldn'ts" around food in my dieting and eating disorder days. I let outside forces decide what I would eat, instead of trusting myself to know best. When I did that for a long time, I was really out of touch with what felt good in my body or what my body even wanted at any given time. I had to put more energy into stopping and listening than I have to do now. A more open, accepting, and learning-oriented way of eating is something that I do pretty naturally now. I believe we can all get there with intention and practice.

Step 9

I've said that the 10 Steps outlined in this book are not linear. They also aren't easy, particularly if you've spent a lifetime dieting or struggling with an eating disorder or having a shaky relationship with food. I encourage you to prepare, choose, and eat foods with love and intention. You will feel cared for in the act of eating as you do this. Move your body with love and intention. Your body will thank you—even if it groans a bit when it starts rolling in a new way. I see it happen over and over again, and it's why I still love the work that I do after twenty-two years. A simple act—eating food—makes us feel cared for and frees us up to make other choices that bring our lives richness, fullness, and meaning. I invite you to discover a way to eat that makes YOU feel your best and allows you to get on with living your very own fantastic life.

Resources and References

Koenig, K. *Starting Monday: Seven Keys to a Permanent, Positive Relationship with Food*. Carlsbad, CA: Gurze Books, 2013.

Melina, V. and Davis, B. *The New Becoming Vegetarian: The Essential Guide to a Healthy Vegetarian Diet*. Summertown, TN: Healthy Living Publications, 2003.

Spear, N. *Healthy Gut, Healty Life*. Asheville, NC: Wellness Ink. 2017.

STEP 10

Know the Company You Keep: Building a Support Tribe

You are a child of God. Your playing small does not serve the world. There is nothing enlightened about shrinking so that other people won't feel insecure around you. We are born to make manifest the glory of God that is within us. It's not just in some of us. It's in everyone. And, as we let our own light shine, we unconsciously give other people permission to do the same. As we are liberated from our own fear, our presence automatically liberates others.

~ Marianne Williamson in *A Return to Love*

Y ou have arrived at Step 10, the last step on this healing journey. Always remember that these are not linear steps. You may circle back to work on Ditching Dieting (Step 1) when you notice that the latest food craze has you stuck in that diet mentality again. You may circle back to Body Acceptance (Step 2) when you receive an unkind comment from a relative who points out that you were thinner last year. You may circle back to Awareness (Step 3) when you notice that you are out of touch with your hunger and fullness, mindlessly eating while you stress over a project. This journey is also not one with a predictable end point. We don't just wake up one day having an ultra-healthy relationship with food like some of us did when we were toddlers and food was one of the many pleasures of life. (And if you didn't even make it to toddlerhood with a healthy relationship to food, well, then this process might take even more work and time.)

I call myself "recovered" from an eating disorder because I believe in full recovery. I am not saying that in the last couple of decades I have never had an ill thought about my body. It does not mean that I eat mindfully and with love, attention, and intention every meal. "Recovery" means that I do occasionally use food to manage stress or forget to eat when my body needs to once in a while. "Recovery" means that I am still human and not perfect. I don't always make eating and self-care choices from a place of balance, but I strive to. Most of the time, I don't beat myself up when I'm off balance. Writing this book has been a journey of learning how to manage a different kind of stress: Deadlines, staring at a screen for extended periods of time, and sitting on my butt for long hours. These are not on my "favorite things" list, and I have found myself out of touch with my body and its needs from time to time while embarking on this intensive writing project for the first time.

When we have an intention, we can often find that we go off course and need to circle back. It's the nature of the mind to wander, as most practitioners of meditation know. **It's human** nature to find ourselves back in familiar, well-grooved patterns when we are tired or under stress. In these instances, we can remind ourselves that we are human and reset our intention to work on the practices that bring us to a healthy relationship with food, our bodies, and our selves. And there is nothing that helps to remind us of how human we are then to spend time with other people who are on the same path.

I've been doing individual nutrition therapy to treat disordered eating since 1997, but I've noticed some of the most profound healing in the small groups that I've been running in only the last several years. My **No Diet Book Clubs** are small, therapeutic book clubs in which members read books together and support each other on their journeys toward recovery from disordered eating of all types. They are little support communities, and it is my honor to witness and facilitate the healing that occurs during these meetings.

Disordered eating can be isolating. Although many of us struggle with feeling balanced around food, it's not something that we often share with others. I take that back. We do sometimes talk about the latest diet that we're on or the food we're eliminating this week and how good we feel about it. But how often do we share the challenge of moving toward accepting a body that we have loathed for so long? I hear many women bashing their bodies in store dressing rooms. I've heard young girls do it in the back seat of my car. (Much to the chagrin of my preteen daughters, I speak up about it.) Why can't we support each other in respecting and loving our unique, diverse bodies that do so much for us? Why can't we share the often-bumpy journey around learning to take good care of our bodies and selves? How often do we share the pain of finding ourselves eating compulsively again—or the significant pain underlying that compulsive eating?

Sharing our grief, sadness, longings, loneliness, and anger is not easy. Many of us, particularly those raised female, are trained to put on a happy face and act like everything is "fine." Talking about how lonely we feel at night, or the grief around letting a dream go, or the loss of a loved one makes us vulnerable and feels risky. Over the years, however, I have learned that the biggest risk is to "stay small" (as Marianne Williamson so poetically said in the quote that began this chapter). When we stay small and say nothing, we engage less in our truest life, drain our vitality, and miss out on community. **We were all put on this planet together, and we benefit most from living when we find ways to do this messy "life" thing together.**

And you don't have to be an extrovert to take advantage of what I call **building a tribe.** First, take time to know yourself better and discover how much social engagement—balanced with time to yourself—you need to thrive. Everyone is different. There is a continuum with extroverts (who need lots of social engagement and find this energizing) at one end and introverts (who build their energy from time alone) at the other. Most people fall somewhere between the two extremes. When you are ready for social engagement, I invite you to consider the company you keep carefully.

- **Are the people that you spend the most time with energizing you or depleting you?**

- **Do you feel good about yourself when you spend time with the company you keep?**

- **If you were to form a "tribe" that would support your healing around food, body, and self, what would those people be like?**

If you ask my group members, I think you'd find that many of them are surprised to have befriended each other. Many of them come from different walks of life and have different life experiences. What they have in common is a desire to dig deep to get to the core of their food issues and recover from the inside out. They are not looking for a quick-fix diet, though they admit to sometimes getting sidetracked by the internet or the latest fad. They are trying to heal and change their strategies for dealing with life's stresses to something more useful and self-loving than starving or purging or binge-eating. They want to feel connected to themselves, to each other, to their lives. They aren't afraid to talk about the times when the messiness of life makes them want to disappear into their food habits again. They care enough about themselves and each other to show up and support each other's journeys. I always go home from work on my Book Club days buzzing with inspiration. Most of my writing of the last five years has been fueled by the energy of these communities. I honestly believe that we heal not only in the quiet of our own hearts, but in shared life experiences.

I was fortunate enough to have unconditional love and acceptance around me when I recovered from my eating disorder. It allowed me to find my truest self and learn to love and accept it, flaws and all. At first, I couldn't fully take it in, but when those around me kept modeling love and acceptance, I finally decided that I could love and care for myself, too. Then I began to eat with balance, curiosity, and common sense. **When you aren't trying to fix yourself, food can become pleasurable and life-giving again. You don't want to put anything into your body that will make you feel lousy, tired, and uncomfortable if you love yourself. You won't want to feel depleted and hungry if you are treating your body and mind with respect and care.**

The most important pieces of having a healthy relationship with food, as I see it, are these:

- **When you are hungry, check in, and eat what you are hungry for.**

- **When you aren't hungry, but you feel drawn to eat anyway or manage your food in some way (via a diet or other food prescription), check in, and notice what you are feeling and needing.**

- **If you notice your feelings and you need something, try to give yourself what you need. If not, make a request of your tribe to help you meet that need.**

An example of that last bullet point is when Mary opens the cupboard to look for some cookies when she's not hungry but then pauses. She checks in with herself and notices that she feels sad and tired. Lonely, in fact, after a long day. She connects this feeling to an underlying need for meaningful connection. She tries to connect with herself first and provide some soothing, putting her hand on her heart and taking some deep, nourishing breaths. In that moment, this gesture feels helpful enough to keep her from eating, but she still feels that her need for connection is quite strong. She reaches out and calls someone in her support tribe, noticing that the act of asking her friend to listen to the story of her hard day helps meet her need for connection so much better than the bag of Oreos ever could.

It's sometimes hard to find other ways to manage emotions and losses and the messiness of life without using food—either under- or overeating. But finding those other self-caring strategies brings food back to the life-giving, nourishing experience that it was meant to be. And having our non-hunger needs met entirely by ourselves and by the requests that we make to our tribe and environment will then lead to nourishment at an even higher level. It's certainly okay to value health and nutrition. We've learned so much from this field of study. But let's put food back in its place and get on with the rest of our fabulous, miraculous, and, yes, rather short lives.

Dieting and disordered eating can be a way to distract us and keep us from being in touch with uncomfortable feelings. If we aren't going to diet, obsess, and focus on counting calories or restricting anymore, then we are probably going to feel a lot. If we aren't binge-eating and beating ourselves up for doing it, then we might have to face other things that we don't like about ourselves. We need to learn how to accept those feelings. It's important to learn how to tolerate difficult feelings and meet our own needs, but nothing helps more than having a tribe of people who can tolerate those feelings along with us. This tribe might include a therapist, treatment team (psychotherapist, nutrition therapist, medical doctor, movement therapist, psychiatrist, etc.), support group, women's or men's circle, online community, or self-made recovery tribe.

> **Are you living life on your terms, making your own choices? Do you consult with your "team" of loved ones or advice-givers around you, considering their needs and ideas along with your own—or do you give up your own needs for the team, doing what you think you "should" do?**

In my experience, healing a relationship with food is composed of the slow, hard work of changing habits and thought patterns, and no quick-fix nutrition solution will do it. **Trust yourself above all else.** Don't forget yourself when trying to be part of a community, family, or workplace. Feed yourself well so that you can move through life the way you want to: With strength, courage, and not overly influenced by your tribe. Life can be a challenging journey. Appreciate your growth, your unique gifts, and the way that taking good care of yourself helps you move through your unique life with grace. You will truly be a better tribesperson if you are taking good care of yourself first.

I believe that the "last frontier" of healing your relationship with food, body, and self is knowing and asking for what you need. This requires using your feelings as guides and developing successful strategies for getting your needs met. This is the "self" part in the healing work. That said, it's not something that we do outside of community with others. We are the only ones who can know and meet our own needs, but we also need to be able to make requests of our tribe at times to help us fulfill our needs. Keep in mind that your tribespeople also have needs and might not be able to meet your requests, but please don't feel shy about asking! If you are as ready to hear a "No" as you are a "Yes," then that's a clear, honest, loving request.

Remember those Universal Human Needs at the end of Step 7? You may be looking for Connection, Calm, Spaciousness, Love ... Remember the example of Mary, who turned to food because underneath was a need for connection? She couldn't sit around waiting for someone to show up; she had to meet that need by reaching out to a tribe member. Once she had her friend on the phone, she asked for what she needed. "Would you be willing to spend a few minutes listening to what happened to me today? I don't need you to fix it or want any advice; I just need to be heard." This kind of request can take a bit of practice for some of us. Sometimes it helps to let your friend know that you are practicing asking for what you need. You may be surprised at how awkward it feels.

At times, you will want and need something that seems unattainable. When that happens, can you just sit with the sadness and grief and whatever other feelings come up until the feeling passes in that moment? If not, can you use the Compassionate Hand exercise (from Step 8) or your journal or a walk in the woods to soothe and comfort yourself? Or can you call on a tribe member—or the image of a tribe member—to help comfort you in the moment? We all have the same basic needs, though some are more pronounced at different times. We all want to feel loved and to belong. When we know how to meet our needs and make clear requests, we get our needs met more often. When we look at how we respond (or react) when our needs are not being met and identify those feelings, we understand ourselves better. When we get our deep, core needs met most of the time, then we don't have to use food (the symbol of all needs from day one of our babyhood) to negotiate them. Does getting thinner give you the belonging that you long for? (Some women find that it isolates them from their jealous friends and makes them feel "checked out" at dinner gatherings. Not exactly the desired outcome.) Does overeating actually give you the pleasure that you want in your life? (Maybe not when it feels lousy in your body afterwards.) Understanding why you use food—under-eating or overeating—is part of the journey.

Sharing your story and your journey with others also reduces shame and promotes self-acceptance and hope. We can all use a little less shame in our lives. Our world could use a bit more acceptance and hope. I see this in my work with recovery groups all the time. If we can encourage acceptance and hope for each other, then we make the burdens of our journeys a little bit lighter. Clients shared that, when I finally "came out" about my own history of bulimia and restrictive/binge-eating, it was helpful. They understood why I seemed to really "get" them, and it gave them hope that recovery was possible. I don't talk about my own recovery in client sessions; that is their time. But if they want to read a bit about my own thoughts about the journey as a recovered person, it's available. When I lead groups, I do so as a human being who has the same life struggles as the group members. We are all just trying to do the hard thing of living. It seems much more tolerable to do it together. **I consider myself to have a healthy relationship with food, my body, and my self, but that doesn't excuse me from the hardships of life. My recovery does, however, free me up to deal with life's challenges in ways that are more care-taking.**

Sometimes we are helped by support and encouragement from outside ourselves in this recovery process. If you have a trusted therapist, nutritionist, or friend who can assist you on this journey, then you have a powerful ally. Show them this book, and describe the non-diet, self-nourishing way that you are trying to approach food in your life. Tell them that even though your steps may be counter to the popular diet and health culture, you need their curiosity and support—not judgment or advice. As you are learning to be curious and not critical of yourself and your choices, you will do best to surround yourself with those who can approach you the same way. Practice the line, "I don't want to talk about your diet right now. I'm working on listening to my body and nourishing it differently." Educate your health practitioners about Health-At-Every-Size (HAES) and intuitive eating. **Above all, practice and model self-compassion. It's contagious.**

Let's review these nonlinear healing steps. Visit them over and over again until you don't feel the need to anymore. Remember that this is a process that unfolds over time, as you get to know yourself better, understand the feelings beneath the food behaviors that feel unbalanced, and build new skills to help you deal with feelings and meet your needs. At the same time, you will discover the way to eat that supports you on your life journey. You won't let anyone else's ideas about what to eat take you away from listening to your body, which ultimately knows best.

STEP 1: Ditch Dieting for Good

STEP 2: Body Acceptance, If Not Love

STEP 3: Awareness Before Action

STEP 4: Body Trust and Deep Listening

STEP 5: Mindful Eating and Nutritional Common Sense

STEP 6: Conscious, Joyful Movement

STEP 7: Values Clarification to Live a Life You Love

STEP 8: Sustaining Self-Care Practices

STEP 9: Developing a Self-Connected Eating Style

STEP 10: Know the Company You Keep: Building a Support Tribe

I invite you to find the pleasures, the activities, and the people who nourish and ground you. With love and attention—sometimes with hard work and over time—food will fall into a place of balance in your life. You can enjoy and take care of your body, mind, and soul with food, but it won't be the only way you nourish the moments that make up your life. Lastly, please don't be afraid to share the discovery. Today, more than ever, we need to inspire each other with our self-kindness and healing instead of bonding together while we put our bodies and selves down.

I believe that, deep down, we all want to see and appreciate the beauty in ourselves and in all of the unique beings around us. What an amazingly diverse bunch of humans we are with different eating styles, movement styles, and priorities around self-care. We all have different feelings, thoughts, and needs. Let's gather together and both honor and appreciate ourselves as individuals, as well as honor and appreciate our interconnected souls. In doing so, we deeply nourish each other in this shared life journey.

Acknowledgments

I feel much gratitude and humility. I could not have written this book without my extraordinary tribe.

I give so many bundles of thank yous ...

To my clients, many of whom allowed me to share their stories. You inspire me more than you know. Witnessing your hard work and dedication to finding your truest selves is a great honor.

To my teachers and mentors along the way, including Lisa Pearl, Linda Gelda, Wyoma, Deb Goldman, and Margie Schaffel. Other friends and colleagues who inspire and support my creative expression include Lauren Manasse, Mary Ross, Kate Leber, Matthew Packwood, Julie Corwin, Marci Evans, Liz Fayram, Anna Sweeney, Sarah McAllister, Sarah Patten, Beth Mayer, Hannah Saxe, and Sarai Logue. I couldn't do quality work in this field without all of you.

To those who gave their time and attention to review the manuscript and provide valuable feedback, especially Nicole Spear, Kate Leber, Kathy Silva, Lynda Goldman, Marci Evans, Lauren Manasse, and David Sharpe.

To Michele and Ronda of 1106 Design, Lynda Goldman of Wellness Ink, my writing buddy Nicole Spear, and the rest of my book-writing tribe, for giving me the encouragement and accountability that I needed to get through the process of birthing this book.

To all the wise people quoted in these pages, too numerous to list again here. I particularly appreciate esteemed authors Tara Brach, Susan Kano, Karen Koenig, and Jessica Setnick who took the time to read and heart-fully endorse *Nourish*.

To Kyla for brilliantly suggesting the one-word title on a day when she was home sick from school with me.

To Patty James for giving me the inspiration for the No Diet Book Clubs, which ignited the writing of this book.

To my big, loving family, especially Mom, Dad, Nana, Joe, Amy, Emily, Peter, June, and John. Your steady presence and loving support is both incredible and sustaining.

In loving memory of two Grampys and one Nana who always encouraged my curiosity and spirit.

And most of all, to Ava and Kyla for making life sweet, meaningful, and full of love and learning. I couldn't have written this book or have dug deeply into my own messy and amazing life without your acceptance, humor, curiosity, and spiritual teaching.

About the Author

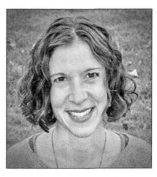

Heidi Schauster, MS, RDN, CEDRD-S is a nutrition therapist, certified eating disorders dietitian, and consultant with over 20 years of experience. She is the founder of Nourishing Words Nutrition Therapy, based in the Greater Boston area, and an instructor in the Eating Disorders Institute graduate certificate program at Plymouth State University in New Hampshire. Heidi is a Health-at-Every-Size (HAES) practitioner who encourages embodied eating and living for all. In addition to individual nutrition therapy, teaching, and writing, she facilitates the No Diet Book Clubs and supervises other dietitians—locally and virtually—who treat clients with disordered eating. Heidi is a lifelong dancer, bumbling gardener, stilt performer, and the proud mama of twin teenagers. Heidi and her daughters enjoy most food that is lovingly and consciously prepared, especially if it is followed by a dishwashing dance party.

http://anourishingword.com

Contact

http://anourishingword.com

If you liked this book:

1. Please join my mailing list by adding your name and email address on my website. You will receive nourishing words seasonally as well as information about in-person and online support related to the Steps outlined here.

2. Please review the book on Amazon. It takes only a couple of minutes, but it helps get this book into the hands of others who might benefit from the work.

Thank you so much!